MAY 15, 2016

Gwen,

'I am support, patience
and faith continue
to move. Nature's
Nurse team

Breath of Life

forward...

.. step by step...

towards international

success;

Thank you!

Happy Birthday!
90!

BREATH OF LIFE

The Vital Role of **Red Mangroves**
for **Human** and **Planetary Health**

TED ANDERS, PHD & RESINA KOROI

Foreword by Jean-Michel Cousteau

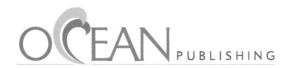

Ocean Publishing
P.O. Box 1080
Flagler Beach, FL 32136-1080
www.oceanpublishing.org

Ordering Information:

Quantity sales: Special discounts are available on quantity purchases by corporations, associations, and others for fundraising, corporate gifts, and other special projects. For details, contact the publisher at the address above.

Orders by U.S. trade bookstores and wholesalers. Contact Independent Publishers Group (IPG), www.ipgbook.com, (800) 888-4741.

Printed in the United States of America
ISBN 978-0-9908431-0-8
First Edition
10 9 8 7 6 5 4 3 2 1

Note: Because Fijians learn English as taught in the United Kingdom, some words in this book may be slightly different than American English. Examples are rhisome/rhizome, metre/meter, etc.

CONTENTS

FOREWORD

Jean-Michel Cousteau
Ocean Futures Society
Santa Barbara, California

DURING MY CAREER I HAVE LED MANY educational excursions in the tropics. Participants are always excited to explore the wonders of the coral reef but my suggestion to venture into the mangroves has had a far different reaction. A typical comment is, "Why go into a swamp of stinky mud, infested with bugs?" My response is, "Well let's see if what you imagine is really true." Often at the end of the excursion people comment that the best part of their adventure was exploring the mangrove ecosystem, partly because what they experienced was so unexpected. Fortunately the prejudice about mangroves is diminishing and I am pleased to see that Ted Anders is continuing that switch from societal ignorance to appreciation.

I was first introduced to the wonders of the mangrove ecosystem in the 1940s when I was in Madagascar. My dad, Jacques Cousteau, took me snorkeling among the labyrinth of mangrove trees and I discovered an amazing, almost bewildering, variety of creatures. I didn't know any of their names but I had the feeling of being in a jungle gym populated with science fiction creatures. I have since learned that I was in nature's nursery where birds come from thousands of miles away to feed and nest, and where the juveniles of fish that live miles away on a coral reef grow up safe from predators too large for the spaces between mangrove roots. Yet this ecosystem is not only a nursery but where many residents filter and clean the water, recycle nutrients and who create an amazing food web extending from far inland and great distances at sea.

Mangroves are also extremely important to the hydrology and geology of coastal regions. Mangroves are territorial plants that evolved to tolerate and even thrive in seawater. The various species of mangrove trees create forests of the sea and do what trees all over the world do – they protect the ground from erosion. Many species, particularly the red mangrove, have prop roots that reach down into the sediments to stabilize and secure them from currents and wave action. This is good for the mangroves and also good for the coastline. Because of their tenacious grip on the bottom and their dense coastal populations, they prevent coastal erosion and reduce the impact of storm surges and even tsunamis on coastal communities. Not only do they protect coastlines but they build coastlines. As the prop roots extend down into the sediment of shorelines they slow the flow of water. This causes sediments suspended in the water to settle out and thus the mangroves actually create land.

Now we are learning that red mangroves may even have medicinal benefits. I applaud Ted and Resina for paying attention to what some village people have known for generations and conducting serious investigation into the biologically active chemicals of red mangroves that appear to have curative properties. I'll let them tell the story of their fascinating journey into the world of red mangroves.

Jean-Michel Cousteau
President, Ocean Futures Society

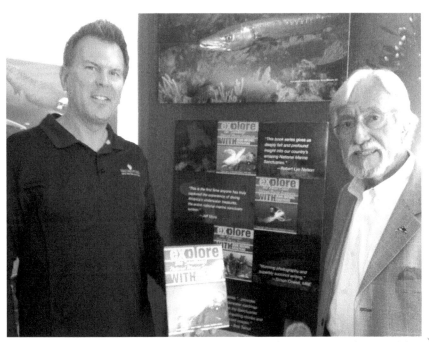

Ted Anders and Jean-Michel Cousteau at the OFS Office in Santa Barbara, California, discussing Cousteau's books on exploration of the oceans and the importance of red mangroves in ocean ecosystems.

INTRODUCTION

Greg Cumberford
President, Bent Creek Institute
Asheville, North Carolina

AS YOU OPEN THIS BOOK AND READ these words, you are breathing. Your diaphragm and lungs are coordinating together perfectly, rhythmically, and for the most part unconsciously, to supply your entire body—your bloodstream, your brain, your innumerable cells and connective tissues—the oxygen it needs to respire properly. Deny yourself breath for anything more than a few moments and your physiology reacts immediately to correct for the imbalance. Deny yourself breath for longer than a few minutes and your life is either severely impaired or it is probably over.

How did we humans and every other living being that respire for its very existence enter into this dynamic interplay of sunlight, atmosphere, ocean tides, and green photosynthesis? It is an ancient primordial story whose pivotal events took eons to unfold: the conversion of Earth's earliest liquid ocean composition from a toxic stew of sulfuric acid and methane to life-bearing sea water; the emergence of the earliest bacteria; the arrival of photosynthetic organisms that could convert sunlight into carbon-rich sugars that could be stored in their cells; the dawn of mobile organisms capable of feeding and digestion; and—eons upon eons later—the emergence of animals with circulatory systems capable of respiration. Like you. Like me. Like every being that swims, crawls, climbs, or walks on this Earth.

To have an atmosphere that supplies a perfect balance of oxygen, nitrogen, and other trace gaseous elements to our lungs required billions of years of green cells from the plant kingdom to respire... to consume carbon dioxide from the air and replace it with oxygen. This fantastically slow, steady, and immeasurably complex process, by which it became even possible for the earliest respiring animals to develop, and thus the earliest hominids as we did some 4-5 million years ago came from the plants. The blue sky and the deepest azure seas appear to our eyes as they do because of the atmosphere that the plants, from algae to azaleas, have bestowed and maintained for us patiently over eons of time, for far longer than our kind has ever existed.

Imagine for a moment what happens at the cellular level when you breathe. With each breath you take, can you feel your billions of alveoli transporting oxygen to your worn and hungry red blood cells? Can you close your eyes and feel the tidal shift at the peek of each breath, right before your diaphragm expels spent carbon dioxide from your body, only to receive the blessings of another breath laden with life-giving oxygen? If we can slow ourselves down enough for just a few moments to appreciate what is happening inside our lungs, and realize that each breath harbors the dual gift of carbon dioxide given to the plant kingdom, and of oxygen for us appropriated from the plant kingdom, it puts much of the miracle that is life in this biosphere in immediate view—even though we hardly ever "see" the air we breathe.

You may recall from high school biology class what lung tissues look like in cross section. Major lung sections branch off from the trachea and airways, then section off further like broccoli florets, then yet again in an organic fractal pattern seemingly without end until submicroscopic dendritic passages allow for molecular oxygen transfusion into our bloodstreams. A healthy set of lungs is truly a miracle of physiology and, indeed, of zoology—yet something healthy people take for granted, like eyesight, hearing, or taste. Our lungs flex constantly with the tides of inflowing and outflowing air, in pace with our waking and sleeping, our state of calm or exertion, of emotional languor, laughter, or distress. In all states of climate and altitude, they adjust responsively in sync with our body's needs for optimum cellular regeneration. Our lungs are a wondrous and yet basic biological process for our bodies.

When we carry this process from our bodies out to the next organizational level in nature—the ecosystem—we find a startling analogy between our lungs and our riparian estuaries. These are coastal wetlands that form some of the most fertile and fecund nurseries for marine and avian life alike. These are the places that link terrestrial life and marine life in a continuous web, mediated by the tides and by the annual flux of fishes, birds, reptiles, and invertebrates that spawn, grow, and proliferate from these inlets, grasslands, and swamps. Viewed from above, we see in many estuaries some strikingly similar shapes and forms as we see at the organ level in the body. We see quick-moving tidal channels yielding to coves and mudflat inlets. Along the cove shores we see yet further crenulation, exposing the maximum amount of surface area to the influence of the tides, to the inflow and outflow of life-giving nutrients and cleansing water. All around the world's estuaries of the tropics and sub-tropics, we find mangroves—which along with phytoplanktons covering the earth's ocean surfaces and feeding the fish that spawn in mangrove estuaries—form the "lungs of the ocean."

Mangroves are special tropical woody plant assemblages that play a pivotal role in estuarine health. Mangroves are somewhat unique ecologically because they grow in salt-laden soils immediately adjacent to brackish waters, yet they colonize these ecosystems by sending down "pencil" roots from their rising, overhanging branches right into the tidal water. Cumulatively, mangroves actually cause new land formation in estuaries where they appear. Mangroves stabilize soil and prevent coastal erosion, especially during episodic tropical storms that can inundate coastal land and reshape coasts to their whim and fury.

Mangroves typically form an estuary's defense against soil loss while also trapping all manner of tidally-borne detritus in their descending roots, like tines on a rake. These tend to form mats that then trap silt and other fine sediments in the water, filtering it to the benefit of many marine organisms, while also providing myriad local habitats for fish and shrimp to spawn. Over years and decades, the roots are eventually enshrouded in new earth, yet extending their "grasp" over new water by their descending tendril roots. Citing their crucial role in estuarine habitat health, most tropical nations put strict conservation rules in place to protect their mangrove habitats.

Red mangrove (*Rhizophora mangle L.*) has traditionally recognized and clinically remarkable medicinal value, particularly for its anti-inflammatory, anti-microbial, and anti-viral activity—which leads to a range of applications involving immuno-potentiation, oral care, and digestive health, as well as wound healing and anti-aging in topical applications. This book uncovers and links these medicinal activities. From an ecological perspective, this rare combination of activities logically follows when one considers the rather difficult environment in which red mangrove has evolved: baking tropical heat and humidity, poor and thin soils, periodic inundation with salt water, and no seasonal respite from insect and microbial pathogens. Yet in these stressed conditions red mangrove flourishes. To accomplish this feat, the phytochemical storehouse of tannins, polyphenols, phytosterols, and polysaccharides in red mangrove had to evolve and synergize to enable this species to occupy and dominate its niche.

Diversification has also helped red mangrove broaden its portfolio. In the Fijian archipelago, red mangrove is actually a complex of three sub-varietals: samoensis, stylosa, and selala. Each occupies a specific sub-habitat in a given estuary complex. Traditional Fijian people, whose presence in the Fijian archipelago dates back to pre-historic times, came to recognize the value of a hot water decoction (or tea) of dried red mangrove roots sampled from all three varietals of *Rhizophora mangle* for children and adult stomach problems and upper respiratory challenges. Perhaps uniquely in Fijian traditional society, however, women controlled (and still control) the development and distribution of red mangrove for its medicinal value. Tribal values and ethics in Fiji assure a matrilineal succession in ordering daily life at the village level. This means that women control how and when red mangrove can be harvested for its medicinal value.

In Fijian civil society, red mangrove can be legally harvested, but because of the intense sensitivity around potential ecological harm to their estuaries, Fijian women (the traditional "wise woman" healers), with guidance from Ted Anders and Resina Koroi, have developed a fascinating "zoned" approach to red mangrove harvest. This assures that only mature roots are harvested by hand and are cut in a way that stimulates faster re-growth of the roots—much like pruning fruit trees stimulates more branches. Individual mangrove bushes that have been harvested are then left alone for 3-5 years. In this manner, a managed eco-system by local women working in a hand-harvesting mode assure the long-term sustainability of any red mangrove harvest. This sustainable systems approach coupled with the relative isolation of many of the Fijian islands assures that each harvested root is very clean and free of contamination risks. Other tropical nations, such as Cuba, that supply red mangrove roots into topical and cosmetic markets, do not make the degree of eco-social commitments that traditional Fijian society does to protect this incredible medicinal plant's capacity to heal people while nurturing a diverse tropical ecosystem.

As you read this fascinating and unique tale of how Fijian red mangrove came to be recognized and adopted into American and European medicinal uses, please take a moment to breathe! Recognize the profound gifts that Dr. Ted Anders and Resina Koroi have brought forward from their families to yours; from the "lungs of the oceans" to the lungs of the people. This is a truly remarkable and heart-inspiring story of friendship, commitment to a higher purpose, and positively fomenting a responsible self-care revolution.

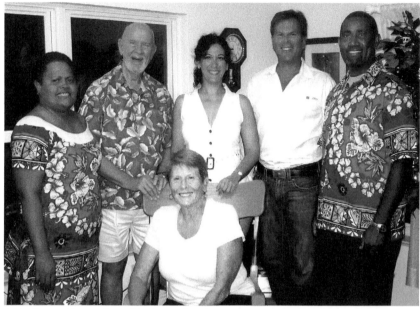

L-R: Resina Koroi, Rev. Charles Anders (Humanitarian Projects Director), Dr. Mary Anders (seated, ensured the company operations were maintained at all key junctures in the company history), Evelyn Hatzigeorgiou (Shareholder, Advisor), Dr. Ted Anders, Semi Dromunasiga (Resina's husband and harvest director).

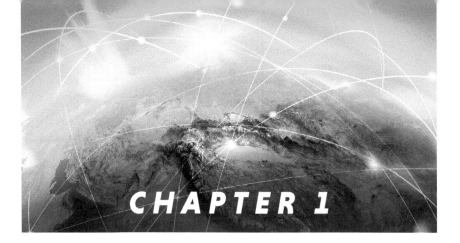

CHAPTER 1

THE FOUNDATION OF
OUR RED MANGROVE
EXPLORATION

Resina Koroi's Perspective

IT ALL STARTED WITH A CHANCE ENCOUNTER with Ted Anders on Air Pacific in 1996. On his way to Australia, Ted was one of 48 passengers on an inaugural flight from Los Angeles to Fiji! A 10-hour flight on a jumbo jet, and we had lots of time to talk to passengers, which got me talking to Ted. At the time I didn't know that Ted was a psychologist, so he had already mastered the art of getting me to share my personal experiences with no hesitation. The conversation led to him asking me about herbal medicine in Fiji.

As soon as he asked me the image of my paternal grandmother, "Bubu Vani," a Fijian term we call our grandmothers, came to my mind and I started sharing with Ted about my childhood experiences when she used to spend the holidays with us. We would trek through

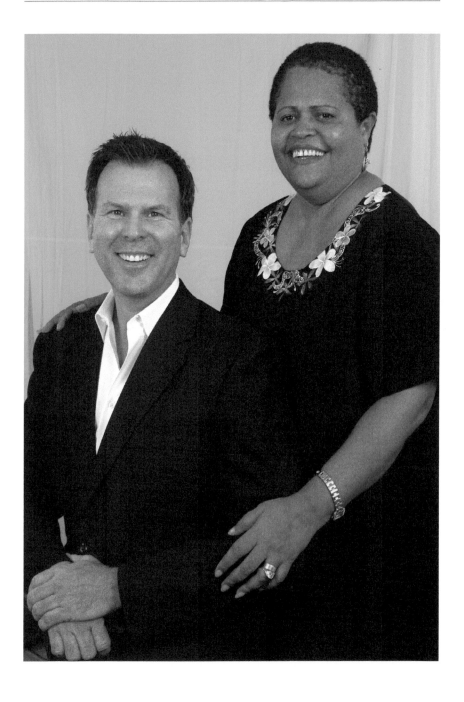

the mangrove swamps where she would explain the medicinal purposes of the plant. When we returned home she would mix this concoction and my six brothers and sisters were all given a teaspoonful after every meal. I went on to share about my experiences with my maternal grandfather, "Tutu Samu," who was also a traditional herbalist and who used to treat the people in the local community. As the eldest of seven children I used to help both collect and prepare the herbs.

Ted Anders and Resina Koroi

Because of our conversation, Ted decided to stop over in Fiji where he met my extended family to learn about the different and plentiful herbal medicines we had in Fiji. At the end of his four- day stay, he took little samples of what he found and prepared them to take home to the States. This book will take you on the journey of discovery with us over more than a decade of exploration, discovery, creation and human service. A story so remarkable, which so profoundly changed the course of our lives, that we never could have envisioned all that would be learned and accomplished.

Four years after our first conversation on Air Pacific, we were underway with the development of a fledgling industry for Fiji. We traveled from island to island building the basics of a new, sustainable botanical agribusiness industry for the economic well-being of the Fijian villagers and the health and welfare of all who will have an opportunity to be healed by the ancient wisdom we re-discovered.

Here's an example of one of our early journeys to establish the world's first red mangrove botanical extract business for dietary supplement consumption in contemporary society. We took a small plane from Suva, the capital of Fiji, to the little island of Kadavu; the ancestral home of my husband, Semi, and I. Upon arrival, we had to trek over a rough mountain mud track to the far side of the island, followed by a grueling boat ride to Namara village where we were to conduct traditional ceremonies and arrange our first harvest contract signing. While there, I saw how the women were struggling to make ends meet and put food on the table. At that very moment I felt a very strong urge to help. I shared with Ted that if we were ever to be successful we had to deal directly with the villagers, honoring their wise traditions, ecosystem, land-owning rights, and human rights. In short, we wanted to lift them from a forgotten economic status to be the proud and rightful stewards of Nature and ancient wisdom they had been since ancient times.

In the village meeting house, we presented the traditional Fijian gifts of kava and a whale's tooth to obtain the blessing and permission from the Vanua (land) and the Spirits of our ancestors. After our presentation, the village choir, who were the current titleholders of the Best Fijian Choir award, sang a beautiful rendition of the Our Father that got our hair standing on ends. We obtained the signatures on our very first agreement and then went to a nearby Home Stay on Galoa Island that used to be a whaling station in the 1800's. The place is steeped in history with the remnants of the colonial station still visible in the overgrown bushes.

I remember standing under the coconut palms on that moonlit night at Galoa and offering up the business to the Divine. That very night, when I went to bed, my ancestors all appeared to me in a vision and gave me their blessings. They advised me to be a good custodian of this gift because it was from the land. The island of Kadavu is still steeped in deep cultural practices and it was only fitting that we planted the foundation of the Company here.

A year passed, and with practically no money in my pocket, I left my job as a flight attendant to get the project off the ground. I had to pull together all resources within my power. With the help of my husband, Semi, and sister, Ann, and Ted's constant support and participation in collaborative planning meetings with all the required government agencies and Ministerial staff, we managed to get the Fijian business established under law. We acquired assigned rights and privileges required to harvest and export red mangrove in an environmentally sustainable manner.

As we obtained more of our exclusive harvest agreements, I became increasingly aware of the importance of this important gift of the mangroves to the villagers of Fiji and to the world. So, we developed a very clear and required educational orientation for the villagers on how to prune the aerial rhizomes, the precursors to the "prop roots" referred to by Jean-Michel Cousteau in the Foreword. We discovered that there was a special way to cut the rhisomes which would allow them to re-grow. We found that when we returned several months later to the mangroves we had harvested, three to four more shoots would be growing from the root we had pruned.

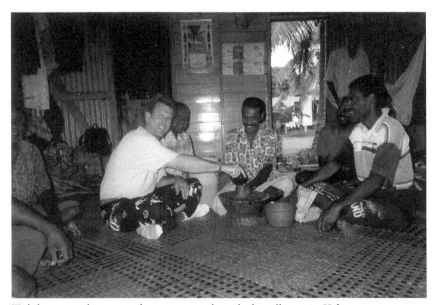

Ted discussing harvest and company goals with the villagers in Kaba.

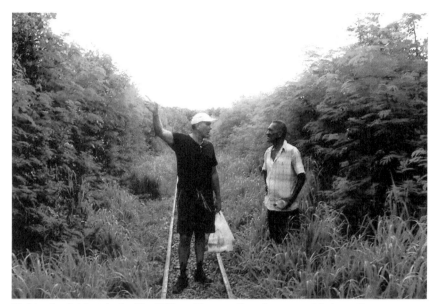

Ted in the field with the Tau Village Harvest Coordinator in Nadroga Province.

Over the years, Ted travelled to Fiji to get more agreements signed and he did motivational talks for the villagers and held board meetings on the progress of the company. One year we held a meeting in the village of Namara in Kadavu, where we had signed our first contract, and we tried to complete all tasks before Ted had to go back to the States. At that time Ted used to spend only one to two weeks in Fiji and he used to come with task sheets which "had to be completed" in the time frame he gave. I could just imagine his frustration when most of these tasks got completed at the time the villagers thought best, which rarely met his timelines!

Ted's Introduction to Fiji Life

One of the challenging parts of working together was Ted's introduction to daily life in Fiji. Our decision to visit my husband's village is an excellent example of how Ted would have to adjust as we structured our business and personal relationship.

In Fiji, especially during the rainy season, the roads are not always usable, so Fijians often travel by boat, even to get from one town to another on the same island. After an organizational meeting, we decided to visit Semi's family in the small village of Daviqele, located at the other end of the island. We figured we would spend a few hours and then return in time to catch the small aircraft we had chartered to take us back to the mainland where Ted could board his flight back to the States that evening.

Little did we know what was in store for us as we set out in a half-cabin 20-foot fiberglass boat. The "captain," who was young enough to be my son, assured us that he was very capable of taking us and he would be able to take us to the airport in plenty time to catch our flight. My sister, Ann, her four children, Ted and Semi loaded onto the boat and we shoved off.

The captain told us it would be a three-hour trip to Daviqele, which we would reach before lunch, giving us two hours to visit and an hour to the airport. All in all, he said we had plenty of time to catch the flight back to Suva at 3:00 pm. When the captain said it would be just three hours to the other end of the island, I was a little skeptical but I thought he knew what he was doing.

Well, the trip to Daviqele took almost four hours, so we decided to spend just an hour with the family, then leaving at 1:00 pm for the airport. The family was overjoyed to see us on this unexpected visit. Everyone thought we would spend the night so they were very disappointed when we said we had to leave in an hour. One of my uncles pointed out that we should leave right away because the tide was going out and we would not be able to travel on the inside of the reef. This meant that the trip to the airport would take at least twice as long as planned.

Promising to come again soon for a longer time, we quickly said our good byes and made our way back to the boat. With the tide receding, we made it only a few meters before we knew it was futile to try to travel inside the reef. The captain, who had been very quiet, announced that we had to go through the passage to the outside of the reef. The waves looked angry and the sound of the surf pounding on the reef was thunderous. I looked across at the captain and saw him nervously looking ahead and saw the uncertainty in his eyes. By now the waves were pounding the little boat and we heard the engine struggling to keep up with the pace of the waves.

I looked across at my husband and something came over me to take control of this situation or something drastic was going to happen to us. With the children screaming and crying to get off the boat I told Semi, "You better get up there and drive this boat or direct the captain or whatever you need to do to get us safely to the airport! You know these waters better than the captain and I'm not leaving the fate of my life to this boy!"

Ted took control of the children; coming up with a buddy system assigning each child to an adult in case of an emergency and allocating an empty 20-liter fuel canister as a floatation device for each pair. In those days we did not think much about lifejackets and other safety issues because we were so used to travelling by boat and many Fijian children know how to swim before they can walk. All of the adults began to reconsider that part of our history! Ted removed important documents and placed them in a plastic bag which he tied to his waist. My sister did the same. We then prayed, so loudly that we drowned out the sound of the waves, which strangely comforted the children.

Semi got the boat under control and instructed the captain how to manage the waves by moderating the engine to fit the force of the waves. The ride was still rough but not as scary as before and the children became much calmer. The one-hour trip had stretched to two and a half hours and we still had a great distance to go even though we could see the end of the runway just inside the reef. So near and yet so far! We knew it would take us another 2-3 hours . . . time we could not afford in order for Ted to catch his flight the same evening! Semi made a suggestion that we would "surf" the boat across the reef to a point just at the end of the runaway where we could run across the tarmac to catch our plane.

With Semi and the captain coordinating the surfing maneuver, the captain would lift the outboard engine and the boat would ride a large wave over the reef. Each adult grabbed a child with their floatation device and prepared for the worst! One! Two! Three and we sailed across the reef on a wave that took us so far inside the reef that the captain was able to power off smoothly! We made our way to the end of the runaway where we saw a tiny speck in the distance coming towards us. We realized it was our plane taking off without us!

We stood up in the boat and shouted and waved our hands in the air trying to grab the attention of the pilot, all to no avail as the aircraft roared overhead! We rushed off the boat and, with children and bags in our arms, we raced down the runaway. When we arrived at the airport the attendant on duty very calmly looked across at us and said, "You're late. Sorry you just missed your flight. We had a high chief here who said he needed to get to Suva quickly on an urgent mission."

Ted, who had been holding it together throughout our ordeal, went "American" right then and there. "What do you mean we are too late? We chartered the entire plane; the pilots were meant to wait for us!" Ted shouted.

"Sorry, sir," replied the attendant softly.

Although we had prepaid for the plane, a local, powerful chief had approached the pilot and ordered him to fly the chief on an urgent mission to another island. In Fiji, when a chief speaks—people listen!

Ted announced, "Aargh! I cannot believe this! You better call the airline company right now and organize a plane to come to pick us up now because I need to catch a flight tonight back to the States."

"Sorry sir," the attendant offered again. "Our telephone is not working. Something is wrong with the wire."

By now Ted was so frustrated he told the attendant to give him the telephone and he would make it work! Pulling the telephone towards him, Ted saw there was only a thin piece of the cable connecting the phone to the wall. He reattached a small red wire and told me to hold it in place while he tried calling. Miraculously, Ted finally got through and a smaller plane was dispatched to pick us up. Ted was able to return to Suva in time for his return flight to the States that evening.

From this incident we learned to allow more time in the islands to accomplish our work. It also made us appreciate the difficulties villagers face when trying to get to the mainland for meetings or to transport harvests in a timely manner. This was a lesson for all of us, but especially for Ted, who has adjusted very well.

Resina's Awareness of Her People's Impoverished Conditions and Her Humanitarian Efforts

We continued our harvest efforts and travelled throughout the Fiji Islands. As we became more professionally and emotionally enmeshed in the village culture and traditions, we learned more about "Wainimate Vaka Viti" (Fijian natural medicine) and also the challenges to contemporary village life. I came to appreciate how much social, economic and physical healing was needed throughout our little country. Buoyed by the resurgence of my spiritual/intellectual connection to my people's beautiful traditions and the natural gifts with which our island nation is blessed, I was led on a very special journey of personal growth and humanitarian service.

Ted's family comes from a 125-year tradition of faith-based social service. His parents, Rev. Charles Anders and Dr. Mary Anders, carried on their parents' humanitarian activities and have served the spiritual and educational needs of thousands of people for decades. They have assisted our companies' philanthropic efforts through their US-based non-profit called, C and M Lifeline, Inc. In 2012, their organization, along with Rotary Clubs in Asheville, North Carolina, West Chester, Pennsylvania, and Dunedin, Florida, cooperated to send 30,000 dried, highly nutritious meals to villages in our Fiji harvest zone whose farms and food supplies had been wiped out by Cyclone Daphne. The meals were flown at no charge by the Fijian national airline, known at the time as Air Pacific, and were received and managed by the national disaster relief organization (DISMAC) headquartered in Lautoka, Fiji.

Our mutual concerns for lifting up the human condition became the cornerstone and core ethic of our companies in Fiji and the US. Certainly, my life path became one focused on service in ways I couldn't have imagined prior to gaining a stronger sense of self-confidence through my dealings with the many chiefs and government leaders in our quest to build a viable national and international red mangrove industry.

For example, in 2004 I volunteered three years of my time at Champagnat Institute, a school for children who had fallen through the cracks of the education system. At least 80% of these children came from single parent families who lived in the nearby squatter settlements. The majority of these families come from the islands seeking the bright lights and a better life for their children. Many children were illiterate and I taught them how to read through cooking in the kitchen during their life skills classes. Most of these students have now become productive citizens.

Reflecting on this situation made me really look at how we could help keep these people in their island villages rather than squatting illegally in makeshift homes on the outskirts of the capital city where they have to live in squalor with no proper living facilities or sanitation infrastructure. Ted and I realized that if we could establish the

Rotary & Women

red mangrove nutraceuticals industry throughout the villages, this new economic sector would allow families to stay in their original homes, earn an income in the villages, and simultaneously care for the precious mangrove natural resource!

Through my work at Champagnat Institute, I joined Toastmasters where a fellow toastmaster introduced me to Rotary International. Its motto "Service Above Self" interested me and their works in the community reflected exactly what I wanted to do personally. So, in 2005 I became a Rotarian. From my association with Rotary, my passion for helping people led me to volunteer at the Kidney Foundation of Fiji. At that time it was operating out of a small office with a registry of people suffering from kidney diseases in Fiji. I helped raise funds from people all over the world to assist the Foundation build Fiji's first-ever dialysis centre. When I left the Foundation to join Rotary's Water for Life Foundation, the centre was in full operation. Little did I know that my volunteering at the Kidney Foundation would later help my aunt when she came from America to Fiji for my mum's funeral in June 2012. My time with the Kidney Foundation also made me aware of the increasing incidences of non-communicable diseases (NCDs) in Fiji and the importance of teaching the citizens of Fiji about healthy eating habits. I became a frequent speaker about these subjects on local talk shows.

In 2007 I became the Projects Manager for Rotary's Water for Life Foundation and was instrumental in providing water to villages that had limited to no access to this basic need all over Fiji. Working with this organization exposed me to the problems grass root people faced and gave me the passion to try to help in whatever way I could to bring this basic necessity to the poor and needy communities of Fiji.

From these experiences I learnt to deal with people from all walks of life, from the most impoverished – seemingly without resources or options to change their life conditions – to the wealthiest and most influential in the country who provided financial resources to my projects. As my leadership role grew in our companies and in my humanitarian projects, my network expanded. I came into contact with caring people all over the world. For example, in 2006 I joined Ted in New York City to participate on several television talk shows to introduce our natural medicinal plants and products. My experience there, and in Washington, DC on the same trip, built my confidence to return to Fiji to speak on behalf of those who are impoverished or those without the resources of life, such as clean drinking water. In fact, I returned to Fiji even more committed to our companies' eco-social sustainable business model, which has become the signature of our activities throughout the Fiji Islands. I will describe our model in detail in Chapter 5. For now, let me share with you some of the most precious moments from our harvests over the last 10 years.

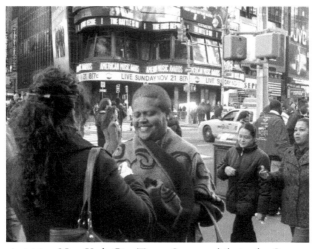

Resina Koroi visiting New York City Times Square while in the States to broadcast the news of the "re-discovered" healing properties of red mangrove extracts on local cable talk shows

So often, we have seen how the lives of vulnerable women have been touched by their ability to provide additional support to their families using the money earned from red mangrove harvests. We have been inspired by children helping their aged grandparents and the church minister demonstrating how to "harvest for the Lord" by bringing in the largest harvest in the village of Bau, the home of ancestral chiefs to which I have paternal links. The money earned by the minister went towards the repair of the village church.

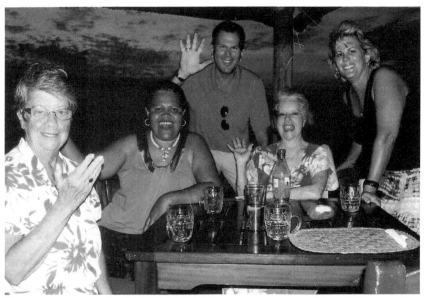

L-R: Beverly McElrath (Fiji McDonald's Franchisee), Resina, Ted, Pat Watson (humanitarian and Beverly's sister, and Becky Anders, Nature's Nurse International's special projects director, celebrating philanthropic project successes at sunset at Vuda Point Marina.

My people have continued to inspire me and I must share from the heart the beauty of our village traditions, many of which could be adopted in "advanced" societies for wealthier communities and balance.

S. Dobey, of the St. Columban's Mission Society, had this to say about the Fijians he encountered during his mission work with local villages: "...there seemed to be something deep and spiritual about Fijians. Perhaps this comes from their closeness to the earth, to water..."

Respect for the land and its tradition is ingrained in every Fijian and this is shown each time there is a kava ceremony asking the blessings and the permission of the ancestors before embarking on any major project which involves the village land or sea.

It literally takes a village to bring the red mangrove to you! Fijian society values the family and everyone takes care of each other. This is especially evident when there is a harvest. The total amount of kilograms of red mangrove needed is divided equally between every home in the village, thereby taking care of the elderly and those who may be incapacitated in any way. The villagers themselves make the decision on how the total harvest will be divided. What works in one village may not necessarily work in another. Every villager takes part in the monthly village meeting where everyone has a say in village affairs and this is also the forum where we, as a company, discuss to some length our objectives before proceeding further.

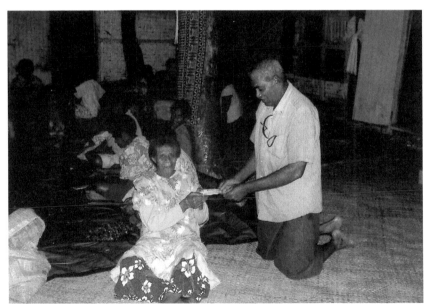

Village Grandmother receiving payment from the village leader in a Nature's Nurse post-harvest payment celebration ceremony.

In the village each person knows their individual role and what they are each responsible for. Respect for each role is paramount. It is communal living where no man is an island. The birth of a child in a village is celebrated as this heralds a new life and a new beginning. Every mother in the village becomes a second mother to the child and it is not uncommon to see the child being passed from one family to another. This strengthens family bonds and eases the pressure off a new mother who can get back quicker to taking part in family and village activities.

Borrowing from each other is also a normal occurrence. When one household runs short of an item, children are sent next door to "borrow."

The village has its own timetable and "Fiji time" is practiced by many Fijians, much to the frustration of foreign visitors who can be kept waiting for services. When Ted first started coming to Fiji, he was always fastidious about time and his appearance, and I used to say to him, "This is Fiji, no one cares what you wear or what you earn. They only care that you will be able to help them in a caring and loving way. You have to be prepared to accept Fijians as they are and not try to change them or their way of thinking. So go with the flow and enjoy the beauty of its people and its culture; it will be less stressful for you."

All these years later, Ted has fully embraced our culture; working hand in hand with villagers and living amongst them, experiencing the daily hardships and struggles they go through and finally understanding what it is to be a Fijian through and through.

During my interaction with villages across Fiji I have found the strength of the Fijian woman to be phenomenal in a discreet and gentle way and this has taught me a lot in my dealings with the village hierarchy. I have found more information about the village politics and beliefs in the kitchen with the women than around the kava bowl with the men. When the earnings from the harvest are received by the women, these directly go for the welfare of the family and that is why it is stressed at pre-harvest village consultations that the women play a leading role in the collection of the product.

The influence of strong women in my family, including my grandmother, aunts and my late mother, enabled me to speak my mind and to be confident in dealing with others. The traditional knowledge I learnt at my grandmother's feet and in my mother's kitchen proved so invaluable in my latter years when I had my children. My son Benedict and my daughter Alexis grew up drinking herbal medicines, mostly one called "Titi," and I believe this is what has sustained them over the years, hardly ever succumbing to seasonal illnesses and other respiratory challenges. Benedict is now in the Special Forces in one of the best military forces in the world. He is a proud husband to Helen and a wonderful dad to our beautiful granddaughter, Eleanor Frances, and adorable grandson, Seth Keverieli Ratulailai.

Alexis was born with physical and mental challenges and had many allergies to western medicine when she was a baby. Her exposure to 'Titi' and other Fijian herbal remedies has made her the strong beautiful 26-year-old she is today, who loves reading, playing computer strategy games and meeting and talking with people from all over the world who frequent our home.

In some Fijian villages, the concept of me owning my own business and dealing overseas with a white American man was foreign for them, so, respecting village protocol of traditional male decision dominance, I have had my husband serve as the company spokesman. This was ten years ago and Fiji has developed so much since then. Still, however, it is often very valuable to demonstrate the equal partnership in life which he and I model for the villages.

Just as I was taken to the mangroves as a child and shown how to prune the plant very carefully, treating the mangrove swamp with respect because it was also a source of food for the family, so the tradition continues today in some of the villages. However, Fiji has also caught up with the rest of the world in technology and my fear is that traditional practices and knowledge will soon be a thing of the past. Hence, my passion in educating villages in maintaining this link with the past and the importance of keeping up with the practice of using herbal alternatives for health.

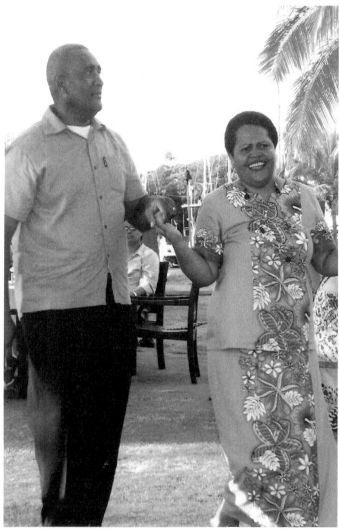

Resina with her husband Semi Dromunasiga who was instrumental in negotiating harvest rights and overseeing harvest production when certain village leaders deemed it inappropriate for a woman, Resina, or an American, Ted, to lead our team.

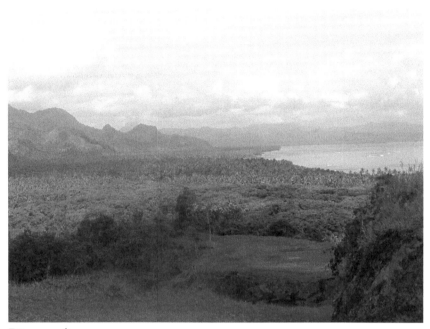

Fijian coastline.

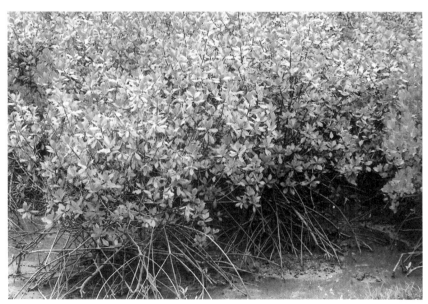

Close-up of red mangrove mangle at low tide.

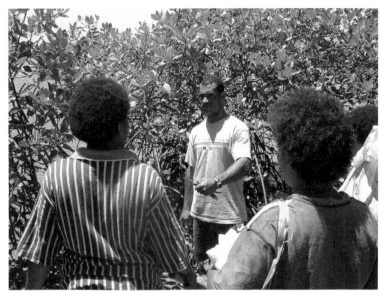

Villagers are taught to harvest according to traditional and sustainable methods.

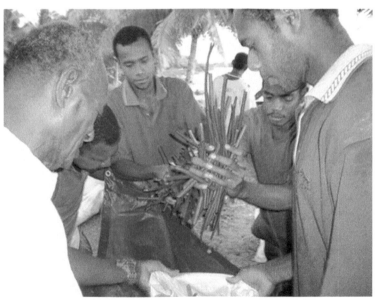

A whole village participates in the complete process of picking, pounding, drying and packing.

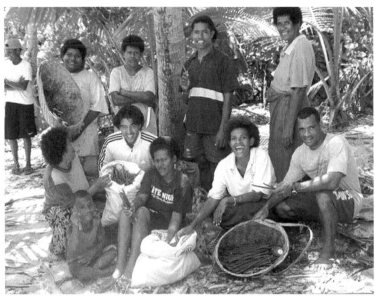

When there is a harvest, an atmosphere of fun envelopes the village as the sound of laughter can be heard everywhere.

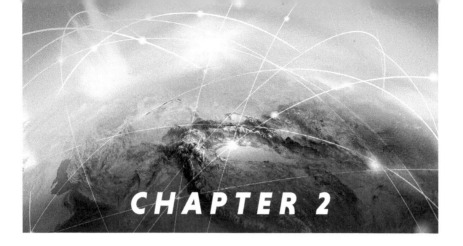

CHAPTER 2

PROVIDING ANCIENT
FIJIAN MEDICINE TO THE
MODERN WORLD

Ted Anders, PhD

ONE OF THE LEADING CAUSES OF DEATH in the United States is FDA-approved pharmaceuticals used according to the manufacturer's instructions and prescribed accordingly by physicians. Our bodies were not meant to attempt healing (i.e. re-balancing) "dis-eased" bodies with only the synthetic versions of plant components. Most pharmaceuticals are modified versions of natural healing plants. The reason they are synthesized is to provide a standardized, controlled product which has a known probability of curing or treating a disease condition. This reason is sensible and necessary. The other reason is that these derivatives of nature can be patented, owned and controlled for billions of dollars in profits. This reason is where the trouble for the consumer/patient begins.

Given the financial and political lobbying power of companies with billions of dollars, a pharmaceutical can become an FDA-approved drug and released into the market with as little as a 35-40% (or lower) efficacy rate. That same pharmaceutical can be deadly to a significant percentage of its users. The consumer is bombarded with advertising afforded by these billions in profits; whether or not the product being advertised is safe or effective for the majority of patients. Today's consumers are awash in a sea of media and politics which can drown them in a wave of greed and ignorance.

We have been created to live in harmony with our green, garden planet which is ripe with healing phytochemicals (the active substances in plants) in all the organic fruits, vegetables and other botanicals. Yes, natural plants must be used in an informed, wise, manner because they, too, can cause harm if misused. However, only the healing claims of natural plant products have been suppressed. Medical claims are made by their pharmaceutical manufacturers for far less effective or even harmful products. Politics of the last century have led to a complete suppression of the rights of natural products manufacturers to make any medical treatment claims. This situation is what leads to consumers being ignorant of the power and relevance of the wise, informed, controlled, use of natural plant medicines.

Our purpose, since our first "re-discovery" of the most ancient medicinal botanical in the world's history, has been to provide powerful, safe, reliable, fast acting "nutraceuticals" (i.e. scientifically analyzed and produced natural medicines) which are so impressive, the consumers – especially leading physicians – are awakened to the wisdom of being healed by nature. In fact, our theme is: "*Health Care Reform is Self-Care Reform…Naturally!*" Our vision is to see a globe of consumers offered a brilliant market menu of the best, safest natural *and* man-made solutions for every disease and for the initial, subtle imbalances in our human body systems which eventually lead to chronic disease conditions.

Initially, we set out to find a natural solution for my daughter, Natalie's, chronic sinus and ear infections because man-made, synthetic solutions were not healing her. So, Natalie's story can serve as a metaphor for the need for substantial changes in our "western" health care systems. Let's look at her story and the amazing discoveries and experiences which resulted.

When Natalie was a pre-schooler, she began experiencing a series of colds which led to sinus infections followed by ear infections so extreme the pus would build up in the middle ear and break through the eardrum. By the time Natalie was seven, she was hospitalized to have her right ear drum replaced. You can imagine how frustrated her mother and I were, knowing that we had followed every pediatrician's and medical specialist's advice. We had used all the pharmaceutical prescriptions and synthetic, over-the-counter products recommended; only to have our daughter end up in surgery. And, following surgery, her infections did not end. We lived through the next two years of her childhood doing everything our pharmaceutically –oriented medical system could do for her. Still, the infections would arise and the resulting pus would break through the ear drums again!

By the time Natalie was nine years old, Resina Koroi and I had met on the now historic Air Pacific flight from Los Angeles to Fiji and on to Sydney. We had extensive conversations about Natalie and our general frustrations with the lack of powerful, natural solutions in our marketplace. Or, rather, the absence of clear medical treatment claims on the available natural products. The FDA and AMA have managed to ensure natural products cannot make any treatment claims; leaving most consumers in the dark about what a natural plant product can do for them. In fact, the following required disclaimer must be included on a dietary supplement package; regardless of how effective the plant product actually is for a disease condition: "This product is not intended to diagnose, treat, cure or heal any disease." Well, if that isn't enough to put off the serious consumer I don't know what is! Nevertheless, our family, like millions of others began to look deeper into natural solutions and discover the truth. Our re-discovery of red mangrove healing medicinal properties is an unusually valuable result.

To get started on our research, Resina and I agreed I would stay over in Fiji on my next business trip to Australia and New Zealand where I was serving as an advisor to entrepreneurial and institutional businesses using my proprietary leadership and management technique known as Customer Driven Leadership™. I arranged to do so and unbeknownst to us, the story of botanical solutions for human health was about to get a major new chapter. On our first foray into the oceanfront forests and tropical mountainside jungles of Fiji, we set out with partial knowledge from Resina's mother's extensive medicinal herbal lore. She and Resina remembered that certain parts of the red mangrove plant were useful for infections. We weren't sure which parts of the plant did what and we needed insights into the specific, ancient understandings of mangrove use and efficacy.

We suspected that many of the older grandmother/herbalists in the villages might still remember and be able to fill in the gaps—although British colonialism and "western" medicine from the 1870s onwards had taken a significant toll on the ancient, indigenous knowledge base. Nevertheless, as we soon learned, some of the natural herbal medicinal practices known in Fijian as "Wai Ni Mate Vaka Viti" (i.e. the healing plant waters of Fiji) were still in use or remembered; especially the unpleasant taste of many plant extracts. (More about the awful tastes in an amusing story a bit later on.) We visited villages miles (and islands) apart from one another to learn and compare answers to our interview questions. As a behavioral scientist versed in anthropological research techniques, I wanted to ensure we avoided biasing the answers we received. So, although we wanted to know about red mangrove (as well as other plants), we did not ask questions about or show interest in, or awareness of, red mangrove as we sat with the grandmothers to interview them.

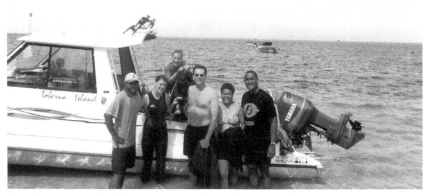

Our boat crew with Ted (in center with sunglasses) beside Resina and Semi, to his left, on one of the original coastline explorations of red mangroves off Viti Levu near Kaba Village.

Rather, we presented a list of disease symptoms and asked which plant or plant combinations were used to treat these conditions. In general, what we learned–and this is a key message–the jungle around the villages and even the fruit trees cultivated outside the bures (the Fijian term for a traditional thatched-roof cottage) are a living pharmacy! The more astute and practiced grandmother/herbalists could walk us casually through the village environs and point out a plant which was known to be effective for nearly every disease state.

My reaction was a complex mixture of deep amazement, further appreciation for Nature and The Divine Source within/behind it all, and a large dose of contemporary western skepticism and socio-cultural arrogance. Given all those reactions, I was vibrantly curious, impassioned and determined to find something that could help Natalie—and also the rest of humanity. After just a few interviews, we were convinced we were on the verge of achieving that goal because of the same experience we had when we asked about treatment for respiratory and immune system challenges.

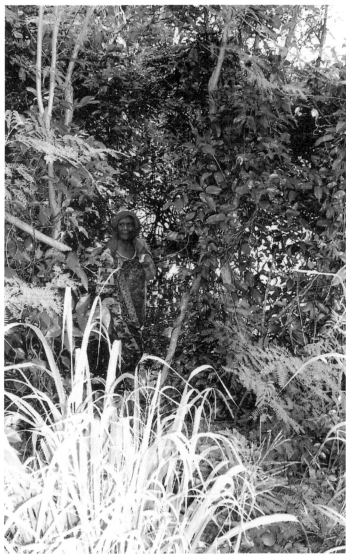

Village grandmother strolling among her natural "pharmacy" from which so many healing solutions are available.

We presented the list of symptoms associated with the common cold and flu and mentioned the related sinus and lung congestion. Without exception, in every village, there was at least one grandmother who walked us over to the nearby oceanshore or riverine mangroves and pointed to the aerial rhizome. The aerial rhizome are the hanging aerial sprouts extending from the branches which eventually grow down and touch the sand or mud soil to become stabilizing roots and a safe haven nursery and home for marine fish and wildlife. The grandmothers showed us which part was the most potent with regard to medicinal properties and showed us where to cut it so that we could prune the plant; not destroy it. We realized that if what we were being told was true, there was a possibility of bringing forward a reliable nutraceutical in an ecologically sustainable manner. However, realizing such a vision was yet a long way off from these first sloppy, mud-encrusted wallowings through Fiji's mangrove swamps.

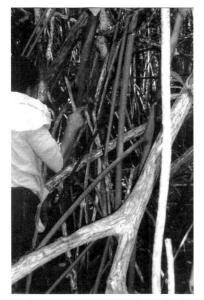

There were many practical steps (and, as yet unknown to us, more than a decade of research and millions of dollars of investment ahead) which had to be taken just to determine the clinical efficacy of the medical claims the grandmothers were making. Not to mention creating a legally compliant, good tasting, marketable product to help humanity in general. So, the first practical step involved Resina and me, followed by trusting family and friends, actually using the mangrove medicine our-

A dense outcropping of aerial rhizomes which eventually grow in a thick "mangle" down and touch the ground to become the root system of the mangrove forest.

selves to convince us that we were really on to something worthwhile. We asked one of the village ladies to make us some of the mangrove tea and we drank it. Dirty, tepid dishwater with an aftertaste of bitter mud describes fairly accurately the perceived message our taste buds sent to our brains. However, we knew that root-based naturals often tasted very "earthy" and our experience was to be expected.

As the lead "western" guinea pig in the group, and the one who was keen to discover a resource and help "save the world!", I volunteered to take some dried mangrove rhisomes back home in a zip lock baggy to make the tea potion made of crushed, boiled rhizomes, bark and all. Resina remembered being given the tea as a little girl and she assured me that it was safe for our children. I took her at her word and, with a little bag of red mangrove parts and pieces, I flew home to the States with enthusiasm.

Back at home in Atlanta, Georgia, in our golf/tennis/swim gated community of "McMansions," BMWs, diamond tennis bracelets and rampant skepticism of anything naturally "green" beyond a manicured lawn, the possibility of my wife allowing me to serve my daughter "tea" made from the gnarled, South Pacific plant parts in my little baggy did not look bright. To prove to her that it would be alright, I would have to crush it and drink it myself; which I delayed for a week or so until I had a quiet moment to clean, crush and boil the mangrove into tea. As it turns out, by the time I got around to making the tea, I had retreated to our lake house on Lake Lanier with noticeable respiratory irritation, which usually signaled the beginnings of a respiratory infection so common in the greater Atlanta metro area.

I remember standing at the stove of our lake house boiling the mangrove parts and looking out over the lake thinking what a world away the waterfront villages in Fiji seemed. It was like a magical dream. Well, for me, the real magic moment came when I drank the tea. Within a minute or so, I experienced a wave of vibrating "warm" energy (for lack of a better term) flowing down my trachea and bronchial tubes. It was evident to me that my body was reacting rather quickly to the essence of the plant. I didn't know what to make of it all but I had no adverse reaction. As the evening progressed, I felt better and, by bedtime, felt quite well. (A comparable experience of feeling and "knowing" that a small amount of plant extract is having an almost instantaneous, energetic effect on your body, take a tablespoon of Braggs® Apple Cider Vinegar. The tart "jolt" lets you know something very active has entered your system.)

Before there was a reason to give Natalie any tea, another member of the family experienced a respiratory and immune crisis for which pharmaceuticals were not working fully or rapidly enough. Our family took our niece, Noor Janho, (whose father is a very experienced emergency physician) with us for a weeklong beach trip to The Plantation on St. George Island off the panhandle coastline of Florida near Apalachicola. Noor had been experiencing upper and lower respiratory system congestion (not unusual in Atlanta, as I said earlier) and was on anti-biotics. While we were all concerned for her, my wife Grace, Noor's parents, and I all agreed that she would be better off recovering in warm, salty, fresh air than staying in the polluted Atlanta air. Our decision to bring her along was called into question by Grace and me several hours down the road as we listened to Noor's thick, deep chest congestion through an increasingly insistent cough. We were very concerned and called her Dad, the emergency physician.

Her Dad's judgment was that she should rest at the beach, take her meds, and she would be fine for the week. I don't think he was hearing over the phone the rattling distress in her chest we were hearing sitting next to her. But, we were closer to St. George than Atlanta and decided we could take her to a hospital in Apalachicola, or even Pensacola, if things got worse. Without mentioning it to anyone, I had brought my baggy of red mangrove rhisomes just in case any of us began to experience similar symptoms and might be valiant enough to give my solution a go.

After listening to Noor struggle with that thick, phlegmatic cough all evening through the drive down and then through the night, I asked her the next day if she would drink some medicinal tea if I made it for her. Of course, I called and asked her parents if it would be alright to do so. I explained thoroughly what I knew of red mangrove medicinal traditions and its safe use with children in Fiji. As Noor's trusted uncle, they agreed to support my suggestion that we do this for Noor since she had been on anti-biotics for several days and her condition was worsening.

I made the tea and added a cup of sugar to the pot because I knew there was no way our young American-Arab princess was going to voluntarily drink the bitter, dishwater-like brew. After some urgent coaxing, we got a cup of tea down her in the early afternoon and again in the early evening. One more was accepted at bedtime. To our astonishment, the next morning Noor's chest congestion was virtually cleared up. Her cough was minimal and she was ready to go out and play with her cousins! And she did so enthusiastically. As a supportive measure, I had her drink more tea throughout the second day. For all intents and purposes, Noor recovered completely in less than 48 hours. We had never seen anything like it. Her recovery was the talk of the family all week. And, the recovery of thousands of patients taking our red mangrove extracts over the years since then has been the talk of thousands of families in the USA, China, Australia, New Zealand, the UK, India and the Tibetan refugee society within India. But more on that scope of things later.

After several more family members in the greater Atlanta area, including Natalie, experienced similar rapid, thorough recoveries from colds/Upper Respiratory Tract Infections and flu or flu-like symptoms, it was obvious to me that red mangrove was a powerful, amazing botanical. Clearly, something had to be done to ensure the world would know about this powerful medicinal plant that was essentially unknown in the contemporary medical or herbal nutraceutical fields. In fact, with the exception of just enough reported prior use (such as a natural anti-biotic by the US Army in WWI) to warrant being "grand-fathered" into the list of USDA-recognized herbs of commerce in the United States, there was virtually no research in the global professional literature on contemporary studies of medicinal properties of red mangrove. There were journal articles reporting anecdotal traditional uses of various genus and species of mangrove. However, we could find almost no late 20th century, controlled, medical research or clinical observations reports on red mangrove. Indeed nearly all reports had to do with the ecological and environmental reasons to sustain mangrove forests along the coastlines of tropical and semi-tropical countries. It was as if red mangrove as a medicinal botanical had disappeared from the radar screen of medical science.

We were determined to change the situation. I allocated funds from my thriving international business and government consulting practice to prepare for the establishment of companies in Fiji and the US to take the lead in bringing red mangrove to the forefront of the nutraceutical and medical fields. Before forming companies, however, it was critical to learn more about red mangroves, their sensitive ecosystems, their recognition in Fiji as a reliable healing botanical, and whether or not the rhisomes could be harvested in an environmentally sustainable manner. In short, we had a lot to learn—and mangrove research was not our full time work.

Resina had her own career with Air Pacific airlines and children, a husband, and many nieces and nephews relying on her for guidance, housing and financial support. I had a global consulting practice, two amazing daughters to whom I was (and still am and will always be) completely devoted, a challenging and inspiring former wife, multiple business, personal and philanthropic financial responsibilities, etc. In short, it took a lot of commitment to improving human health care, naturally, to stay focused on bringing red mangrove from the swamps of Fiji to the clinics, pharmacies and homes of the United States. No easy task, let us assure you. Nevertheless, we made a plan and, "come hell or high water," (both literally and figuratively) we have stuck to it since formation of the Nature's Nurse® companies in 2001 in the US and 2002 in Fiji. Our families have been instrumental in supporting us on the journey.

A Decade of Research and Development

Insights from Fiji

Some folks might think we could have gone full steam ahead with chopping up plant parts, drying them and shipping them to the US to make tea and selling it to the masses. However, if we'd done so, we would have gotten about as far as the Fiji Ministry of Agriculture and the Biosecurity Export Office and been stopped in out tracks. Even if we had been able to ship out bags of partially dried red mangrove rhisomes, the US Customs authorities, on behalf of the USDA, would have seized and quarantined our harvest. Re-discovering a nutraceutical botanical for the markets of the developed nations is a complex, detailed, rational set of sequential tasks full of logistical & financial hurdles, legal compliance, multi-cultural scientific teamwork, and dogged commitment to overcome ignorance and intentional resistance.

We began by funding a study through the University of the South Pacific (USP- Suva, Fiji) to learn all we could about the mangroves in Fiji. A team of professors and students went into the field to validate the available "book knowledge" on Fijian mangrove. We learned so much very fast. The mangroves in Fiji are red mangroves (*Rhizophora mangle, L*) and are the same genus and species as much of the mangrove found in the Americas (including Florida where the red mangrove is known officially in the "United States Herbs of Commerce" records as "American Red Mangrove"). The same red mangrove is found in the Caribbean Islands, such as Cuba, and in other parts of the South Pacific, such as Tonga and Samoa. Due to Fiji's relatively isolated ecosystem, two unique varietals known as v. samoensis and v. selala hybridized into v. stylosa. A simple way to think of these varietals is to imagine a rose garden with a wide variety of flowering blossoms in multiple shapes and sizes; yet they are all "roses."

To see what the red mangrove looks like in Fiji, look at the next two photographs. You can also go to "YouTube: NaturesNurse" and see videos of our harvests conducted in the mangrove. It is quite apparent that the scientific term, "mangle," chosen by famous botanist, Linnaeus, when he named and categorized the red mangrove, is very appropriate because the entire coastal tidewater area is a muddy swamp of twisted, interconnected, roots, branches and rhizomes which appear to be all "mangled." It is quite challenging to make your way through the area as the mud sucks the shoes off your feet and the entangled, mangled flora seems to reach out and grab you at every opportunity!

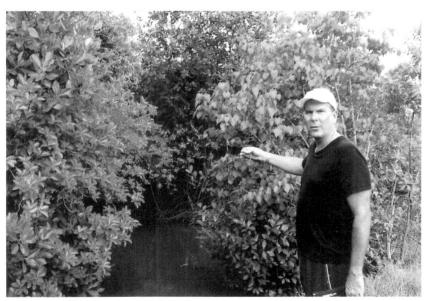

Ted standing on the edge of a mangrove tidal area. One can see the beginnings of the roots and rhizome mangle in the center of the picture underneath the green foliage.

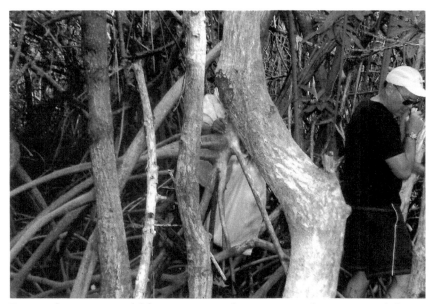

Deep in the mangrove tidal forest one can see how easy it is to become entangled.

Our report from USP also provided us with the area locations of mangrove tracts in Fiji, the total hectares in Fiji (compared to a much smaller number of hectares in Tonga and Samoa), and the ideal, sustainable rhizome pruning harvest quantity per 10 square meters on a recommended three-year cycle. The strong advice from the USP team was to prune the rhisomes at a quantity of 1 kilogram per 10 m2 in year one of a three year harvest cycle and return to that area to harvest three years later; the third anniversary of the original pruning harvest. If done in this manner, the mangrove rhisomes multiply from the site of the pruned rhizome and re-grow reliably and strongly as multiple rhisomes and, eventually, as many roots in the water and soil. Again, see YouTube: NaturesNurse videos showing a harvest video in which the village women demonstrate the pruning practice and we highlight the multiple re-growth of the aerial rhisomes.

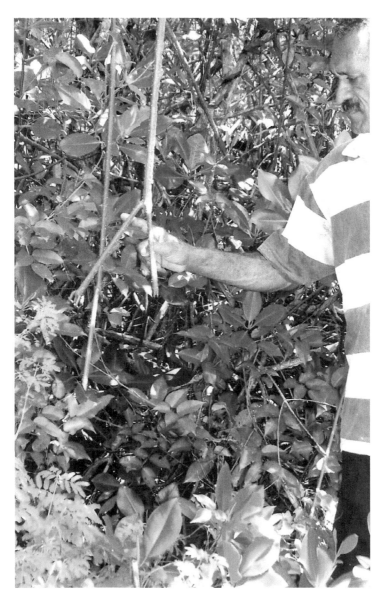

Our harvest manager pointing out regrowth of an aerial rhizome of red mangrove less than one year after our prior pruning harvest.

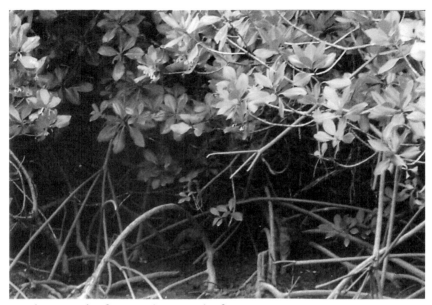

Another example of re-growth as a result of proper pruning.

You might be asking yourself, why is it so important that the harvest be done in this environmentally sustainable manner? As Jean-Michel Cousteau indicated in the Foreword, when mangroves are cut down rather than pruned, their critical environmental management role is removed from the oceanshore tidewater environment and severe ecosystem degradation occurs; often with disastrous consequences for the land, coral reefs, marine life, and humanity. There are so many examples of the negative outcomes which occur when mangroves are destroyed! Here are just a few examples:

- DEAD CORAL REEFS: The coastal soil erodes which destroys the shoreline. The silt is carried out onto sensitive coral reefs and covers the living coral; thereby turning the reef into a virtual "dead zone." This reduces the environments which fish require to thrive

- ERODED COASTLINES: Coastlines which have been stripped of mangrove are more susceptible to damage from high storm tides. One historical example is the US Gulf Coast around New Orleans during the famous Hurricane Katrina. The coast had been largely stripped of mangrove protection so there was no natural wave mitigation provided by mangrove forests. The area experienced the full force of the waves. As "Climate Change" causes rising sea levels (which we have observed personally over the past 15 years in the Fiji Islands) it is essential to coastal regions that they expand their mangrove forests rather than decimate them.
- DECIMATED FISH & CRUSTACEAN NURSERIES AND HUMAN FOOD SUPPLIES: Mangrove tidal zones are the natural nurseries for fish, crabs, and their food chain. When mangroves are destroyed, there is a major reduction in marine life and the related seafood supply to humans in the region. In Fiji, there is a traditional food supply business operated by the village women – the supply of large, delicious crabs to the resort hotel restaurant industry. When mangroves are destroyed near a village, this industry and source of income dies off.
- POLLUTED TIDAL WATERS: Mangroves have an amazing ability to siphon out phosphates and nitrites from agricultural runoff and distribute those compounds throughout their vast root and branch network such that the concentrations in any one part of the plant are negligible.

(Note: University of Georgia doctoral student, Virginia Suttes, is completing studies which demonstrate this ability, as well as demonstrating how the permanently submerged portion of mangrove root systems in the Caribbean host a symbiotic range of life forms. Her research is discovering how the mangrove and sponges exchange these chemical compounds in ways that are beneficial to their respective health status.)

LOSS OF NATURAL MEDICINAL PHYTOCHEMISTRY RESOURCES: We have been leading the way for the past decade in the demonstration of the nutraceutical healing capacity of red mangrove extracts. The synergistic nature of the plant chemical compounds is so unique in nature--and so perfectly attuned to re-balancing "dis-eased" human physiology – that the mangroves must be protected for generations and eons to come. Indeed, as Greg Cumberford pointed out in the introduction, mangroves are the oldest living plant species on Earth in their original form. Clearly, they have a powerful, resilient immune system from which we have so much to learn.

While awaiting the complete results of the USP study, we met with Fiji's Chief Pharmacist, Mr. Peter Zinck, in the Ministry of Health. We interviewed him about the traditional use of red mangrove, "Titi," in Fiji. He researched the ministry's archives and reflected on his own studies of Fijian traditional medicine and gave us an unequivocal positive report on the safe, traditional, medicinal use of red mangrove in a meeting at his office in Suva. He indicated that a hot water extraction method of various parts of the plant had been used for centuries and that the ingestion of red mangrove extracts made from bark, rhizome and mature root was known to be completely safe and non-toxic. Later, we also learned that the US Department of Environmental Protection had announced that topical human contact with mangrove bark and wood particles was considered to be completely safe and non-toxic for humans of all ages. (See 1997 US DEA Report summary. Full reference in Article 15, Appendix C.). Mr. Zinck's information gave us confidence to move further ahead with plans for red mangrove ingestible nutraceuticals. The US Government's parallel position added a plank on the platform of our rationale to create a topical healing lotion made from red mangrove.

So, we had learned from the USP team in Fiji that a sustainable new agribusiness industry could be developed for Fiji. Further, various government and traditional resources deemed it safe and appropriate to ingest and apply red mangrove extracts in, and on, our bodies. As a result of these insights, we were set to tackle the legal approvals required in the United States. Or so we thought, until we ran into a multi-year quagmire of bureaucracy, competing regulatory agencies, partial or mis-information from legal "experts," suppressive self-interested parties, and greedy opportunists in the dietary supplement and nutraceutical industries!

Global Interest and Support

Typically, it takes millions of dollars to "re-discover," register, and develop an addition to a leading nation's approved list of herbal supplements. We didn't have the hundreds of thousands, upwards to a million dollars, to pay all the experts to get us down the path, so we had to employ the "learn as you go" method with a lot of "sweat equity" help by a group of professionals who are now shareholders in our companies. What a challenging, fascinating journey it has been! Here are some highlights along the path:

United States:

Our New York-based lawyer reviewed the national records and determined that red mangrove (*Rhizophora mangle, L.)* had been recognized as an herb used in US commerce prior to the implementation of DSHEA (Dietary Supplement and Herbal Education Act) in the early 1990s. This fact meant that we didn't have to go through the entire approval process from scratch. The costs would have been prohibitive and we might have had to stop there. What a relief we experienced when our attorneys called to tell us red mangrove was a

legal dietary supplement ingredient; although it hadn't been used in
any substantial way since the World War I era.

Colorado: Thanks *Whole Foods*!

We made a plan to produce and sell dried bulk tea made of red
mangrove so that the American consumers' experience would be as close
to the Fijian villagers' experience as possible…naturally! We needed a
first "flagship" test store and an informed, naturally-oriented consumer
market. Whole Foods in Boulder, Colorado, offered to purchase our first
bulk tea samples and host an in-store promotion in the Winter of 2003.
See the first tea bag products as they were being packed and labeled in
Fiji in photograph below. Resina flew from Fiji to the snow-covered front
range of the Rockies in Boulder. She had never seen snow before and her
traditional island costume worn in the Whole Foods store at our display
was quite a contrast to the overcoats and snow boots of the customers.
But, they loved her and several bags of tea were sold that first day.

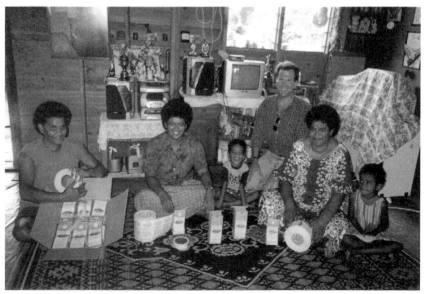

The preparation of the modern world's first commercially ingestible red mangrove tea
product—being carefully packed and labeled in Fiji.

Within days we began to receive phone calls from customers exclaiming their satisfaction with the results of red mangrove tea for their colds and flu-like symptoms. They were experiencing a rapid resolution within less than 48 hours. Our local colleague, Eric Baehr, even received a phone call regarding two elderly sisters in a nursing home; both of whom were in dire straits with viral lung infections. After two days of drinking the tea, each one experienced a major clearing of their lungs and a resolution of the infection. Needless to say we were overjoyed and raring to go. Then we began to hear some suggestions from customers indicating they would like to have the red mangrove in an easy to use bottled extract since some folks don't feel well enough with a heavy cold or flu to get up to make tea.

Those suggestions to make an extract led us into the highly regulated, FDA, USDA, and FTC- compliant dietary supplement manufacturing and marketing arena. Suffice it to say it took years to fund, research, formulate and test a clinically effective, reliable product—a product respectable and promising enough to be adopted by leading physicians. My goal as a scientist, business development consultant, and social entrepreneur was to ensure that every step we took was of the highest standard so that our powerful new products would be seen by physicians as a uniquely powerful "bridge" between their pharmaceutical world and the promising world of nutraceuticals. Remember our original purpose: to awaken the consumer—especially leading physicians—to the solid reality of being healed naturally.

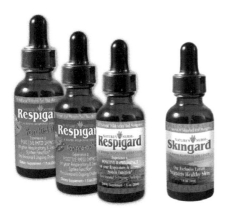

Current Nature's Nurse® Products

England:

As we began to create a serious supply chain business in Fiji to support the anticipated growth of a full-fledged dietary supplement company in the US, we realized that the financial wherewithal to do so was beyond my personal means; given all of life's other responsibilities. Through a series of connections made on my trips as a business management consultant to the United Kingdom, members of our team who were in England with me, Virginia Wadsworth and Denise Stone, were introduced to Mr. William Elmhirst; whose mother was Dorothy Whitney of the New York Whitney family (i.e. Whitney Museum, Whitney Library, and later, The Elmhirst School of Agriculture at Cornell). She had married Leonard Elmhirst, an English agronomist in the 1920s and moved to England to create a rural-utopian, capitalist, cultural revival community. She did so and the result was the amazing Dartington Community and the still functioning school at Dartington Hall.

She had raised William to be highly concerned about the health and well-being of the planet and to have a sensitivity to people and processes in alignment with that general working philosophy. My team members insisted I meet William and he was very amenable to doing so. Nevertheless, it took us nearly a year to get our calendars coordinated so I could accept his invitation to fly down from Glasgow (where much of my entrepreneurial consulting was based). My friend in Glasgow, Janis Sue Smith, flew with me and was witness to the most startling and heart-warming "Spirit Brotherhood" reunion. Although William and I had never met, and he was nearly 30 years my senior, we had an instant affinity and understanding of one another. William's life work for the past four decades had been guided by the theme, "The World Restored Not Destroyed." It was clear our philosophies were complementary and our intentions for "waking" up our species to the importance of honoring God's gifts of Nature mutually impassioned.

Within days of my return to Glasgow, William unilaterally chose to transfer a substantial sum of British Pounds into my account so that I could "do what needed to be done." His input then, and again two years later when he invested in both the Fiji and US companies, were the first non-family funds invested and were essential to our success at the time. I will be forever grateful to William for how he has lived his life and made his decisions based on prayerful guidance from a higher authority.

Italy:

For several years, we continued to develop red mangrove products on a small scale and test them in clinical observations with leading physicians. In the next chapter, I will introduce you to one of the most intelligent, broad-minded, entrepreneurial leading physicians in the United States. His name is Dr. Scott Carroll, pediatrician-immunologist, co-founder of The Atlanta Allergy and Asthma Clinics. Prior to focusing on the clinical observations and the more detailed phytochemistry, I'd like to share with you an experience which occurred in February, 2005 that "sealed my heart" regarding my ongoing commitment to bring red mangrove nutraceuticals to the world. The story I am about to tell you is true and is just one of many nearly miraculous experiences our team has had which motivated us to continue the challenging process of getting a new botanical product into the broader marketplace.

I was in Romania in early February, 2005 investigating the highly successful, all natural "pharmacy" chain called, Hofigal. I met with their leaders and learned how they sourced their botanical ingredients and managed a national chain of herbal apothecaries, as well as an internationally renowned healing spa retreat in Transylvania. I admit I had a little trepidation driving up into the mountains of Transylvania given the lore we have all heard! Upon conclusion of my trip, I flew from Bucharest to Paris and made an overnight stop there. I was scheduled to fly to Atlanta the next morning but experienced what some might call a "divine intervention" instead!

While on the plane from Bucharest to Paris, I read an article in the paper on the health status of Pope John Paul II. The Holy Father had been hospitalized for more than a week and was reportedly unable to return to the Vatican due to ongoing, flu-like, viral symptoms which weren't resolving readily. I said a prayer for his recovery and went on about my schedule after landing in Paris. That night, at about 3:30 in the morning, I awoke with the insistent thought that I needed to go to Rome and take Pope John Paul our red mangrove extract called, "Fiji Tea," at that time.

My more "rational" self-talk said strongly that I needed to get that thought out of my head as it would be impossible to ever get access to the pope. It certainly seemed completely out of the scope of reality that I would ever convince his physicians to let him take an unknown new botanical extract from a stranger. I tried to go back to sleep. But, that "still, small voice" we have all heard from time to time when we are quiet and reflective was persistent. "Go to Rome!" Again, I tried to ignore the "call" and again there was this sense of an overwhelming urgency to go to Rome!

I finally got out of bed, turned on the lights and rationalized that I would call one of the pontifical universities in Rome belonging to the Legion of Christ with which I was loosely affiliated in Atlanta. I said to myself, if: 1) someone answered my call so early in the morning; and 2) they spoke English; I would 3) introduce myself, request to speak to someone who might know if there was any connection the organization had to the pontiff's staff and; 4) if so, ask if they would like me to bring a powerful healing natural medicine to John Paul. I could almost hear the laughter in my head as I imagined the university staff member's reaction to my absurd call "out of the blue."

So, I called and got a heartfelt "*Buongiorno*" and then a rapid switch to English when I said, "Good Morning." I gathered my courage and explained who I was. I informed him I knew some of the Legion of Christ priests in Atlanta (if he was going to need to verify I was not some crazed nutcase with a bottle of poison). And, I said, if by some miracle (little did I know at the moment) he knew anyone who might like me to bring my new, but well documented, anti-viral herbal extract to the Holy Father, I would be willing to do so. I hurriedly said that I understood completely if he felt this was a totally inappropriate call and asked him to feel free to take a moment and reflect on his answer. He courteously asked me hold a moment; which I did. About a minute and half later, the Legion brother came back on the line and in a very calm and confident voice, said, "Please fly to Rome this morning." You could have pushed me over with a feather. "We will meet you at Leonardo Da Vinci airport—just let us know the flight number."

Fast forward to mid-morning in the glaring Roman sunlight (compared to the dreary, foggy Paris early morning) and I was outside the baggage area following two Legion priests who were carrying my luggage to a green Italian sedan. They introduced themselves and suggested we go get a coffee and discuss me, my natural product, my background and intentions further. We did so and in the course of conversation over coffee it was revealed that one of the priests sitting across from me was a close personal friend of John Paul's private secretary, a fellow Pole named, Machek. It was agreed that, after we visited the Legion's headquarters in Rome for further vetting of me, we would drive to the hospital and attempt to get a message to Machek who was with the Holy Father in his hospital suite.

I had no idea the world conclave of the Legion of Christ was being held in Rome that day and the new leader of the order, as well as regional directors, elected and appointed. I was welcomed into the Legion headquarters, ushered into a well-appointed salon, and asked to sit down beside Father Scott Riley, one of the Legion priests from Atlanta!, whom I knew. He had just been selected as the Regional Director for North America! You could have picked up my jaw off the floor. He immediately validated who I was and stated that the priest's home in Atlanta was stocked with my product. Within moments—as my head was spinning—we were on the way to the hospital.

Upon arrival to the hospital it was obvious to me why my extreme doubts about this effort kept re-entering my mind. The hospital lobby was filled with international journalists and security forces. No one was going anywhere near an elevator or stairs leading anywhere near the pope. Or so I thought. Moments later, a priest who knew my hosts, came down the stairs and we caught his attention. Our purpose was explained and he volunteered to carry a message back up to Machek. We were to go have a coffee and await a message. I began to feel like a player in a re-enactment of a Dan Brown novel!

About an hour later, a paper message was delivered to us in the coffee lounge. It read, *"Call me on the following number in our Vatican apartment at 9:00 tonight. I will be at that landline number--if I can get away from the hospital. Machek"*

So, again going with a "flow" greater than any one individual could create, we went and got registered and checked into a convent guest house near the Vatican. We rested until dinner time. At 8:00, we went to a little café nestled on a side street to the right of the grand marble colonnades bordering St. Peter's. The two priests and I had dinner together; with the background thought in each of our minds being a concern as to whether Machek would be able to make it to his apartment next to John Paul's in the Vatican by 9:00pm. The entire trip and related efforts and expenses boiled down to a phone connection occurring that evening.

At 9:00 I gave one of the priests coin tokens for the pay phone across the street from the café. The second priest and I had a pensive moment over coffee while watching and waiting to see if the call was answered. It wasn't. We all retained good spirits and agreed we would call again in 15 minutes. We did so. Again, the call was not answered. After all we had attempted, we agreed it was worth waiting till 9:30 and trying one last time. I reached into my jacket pocket and touched the bottles of Fiji Tea red mangrove extract and said a short, silent prayer. At 9:30, the priest made our last call attempt. If there was no answer, we had agreed I would return to the guest house and fly on to Atlanta the next morning. The second priest and I were scanning the caller's face at the phone kiosk—waiting anxiously for a positive expression on his face. Moments later, his face lit up and he signaled to us that he was connected with Machek!

The next 20 minutes were a blur and a joy. Machek had instructed us to get in our car and come round to the Swiss Guard's gate. At the gate, the guard in full Swiss Army Vatican attire, waved us through and pointed to an underground tunnel entrance. We drove on through the dark tunnel which was constructed of brick in a herringbone pattern. It seemed centuries old and reminded me of Renaissance architecture. But, as I say, the experience was a bit of a blur because of my gratitude and ongoing amazement that the Source of the early morning "Still, Small Voice" had been able to arrange the necessary connections throughout the day and evening in a perfect pattern; all without strain on us and leaving us with a sense of deep peace which passes all understanding. In a matter of moments, our car emerged from the tunnel underneath the Vatican into a cloister-style, residential courtyard which provided the private entrance to the Holy Father's and Machek's apartments.

As we stepped from the car, I stood and stared up at the stars in wonderment and vowed to remember that the forces behind our efforts

Respond to the Rescue!

to bring red mangrove healing nutraceuticals to the world were awesome, indeed. When I looked down, a door into the courtyard opened and an energetic, kind, young man came out to greet us. He introduced himself as Machek's assistant and immediately directed the conversation to the point at hand. He wanted to know the details of the extract and the instructions on how best to provide it to John Paul.

We explained that the product was labeled, "Fiji Tea," and was, in essence, a concentrated version of the herbal tea which the villagers drink in Fiji. Our suggestion, with which he readily concurred, was to simply make cups of herbal tea for the Holy Father. We agreed it best not to suggest an addition to the ongoing, prescriptive treatment by the team of physicians. Because an attempt to explain red mangrove phytochemistry and its infancy in the modern dietary supplement/ nutraceuticals arena would have taken much too long and required a medical treatment team review, we all thought it best to just serve safe, refreshing, energizing tea as a comfort while the physicians continued their treatment protocol.

The assistant asked us to wait a few minutes while he went upstairs to discuss our recommendations with Machek and to deliver the bottles of red mangrove extract; our "Fiji Tea." When he returned, he said they understood what needed to be done. He expressed their gratitude sincerely and presented me with four papal rosaries; one for my former wife, one for me, and one for each of my daughters, Hannah and Natalie. I had no expectations of any gesture of appreciation, so I was deeply moved by the thoughtful act.

My two host priests from the Legion of Christ drove me back to the convent guesthouse. The next morning, they collected me and drove me to the airport. I flew on to Atlanta—having lost a day but having gained an insight into eternity. *In less than 48 hours from our surreptitious courtyard meeting in the Vatican, His Holiness, Pope John Paul ll was fully recovered from the viral, "flu-like" condition and returned to the Vatican.*

Switzerland:

One of the main reasons for sharing the preceding melodramatic story with you is to take this moment to share that Resina and I have experienced repetitive, nearly inexplicable moments throughout the years of our struggle to bring the power of red mangrove to the modern consumer. There were times when we did not have adequate funds to move the company forward. Suddenly, there would be an affirmative reply to one of my investment funding requests. Or, in one instance, at a friend's 40th birthday party in Marbella, Spain, a fellow guest expressed such enthusiasm for our project over cocktails, that I gave him a bottle of our extract for his two young daughters who were upstairs in the hotel sick with colds. They recovered rapidly while we were all still together at the extended birthday bash. He suggested strongly I should come to Switzerland to meet his colleagues who controlled a major "MedTech" Investment Fund. I did so and he, along with two Swiss colleagues, invested their personal funds into the US company. This allowed us to take the companies and product development to the next level.

Fiji:

Experiences like these occurred in Fiji, as well, and memories of them spurred us to continue moving forward in the US and beyond whenever our motivation or focus flagged. Several of these instances Resina has shared with you in Chapter One. Many have had a "spiritual" essence to them; either from a Christian perspective, as with the story in Rome, or clearly influenced by ancient, indigenous island energies. In fact, we initiated our first formal contracts on the island of Kadavu; in a remote village high atop a mountain plateau overlooking the ocean. As we trekked up from the beach bearing our required gifts of honor to the chiefs gathered there to meet us, we could hear the rhythmic pounding of the giant wooden mortar and pestle being used in the thatched longhouse to pound Kava for the upcoming ceremony. The ceremonies are referred to as Sevu Sevu and serve to honor the village, the land, the chiefs, the current residents and the spirits of the departed who continue to protect their lands.

Among our gifts was a sperm whale tooth wrapped in bright orange silk. You can imagine what I thought when I was first told I would need to bring a whale tooth with me if we were to achieve our goal of formal harvest contracts with the chiefs! My first reply was, oh sure, let me just run back to the hotel because I happen to have one in my hand luggage! Seriously, we were meeting with a gathering of six chiefs to request their blessing to begin harvesting the red mangrove *on their island and to do so with deep respect for the ancestors and their medicinal wisdom.* Therefore, a sacred tooth, or "Tabua" in Fijian, had to be obtained. Fortunately, there are keepers of traditions living throughout the islands and we were able to locate a man who maintained a sperm whale tooth for just such ceremonial purposes. We met him at his roadside Shaman hut and paid to borrow the tooth. He wrapped it gently in silk, handed it to us, and placed it in our care.

The next night in the village, sitting alongside Resina and her husband, Semi, after hours of ceremony in Fijian and, finally, English for my sake, the six chiefs nodded to the local village leader who is known as the "Mata ni Vanua." This was their signal indicating they understood all that we had explained and requested. The nod was his prompt to offer the "Tabua" (tooth) to them so they could seal the agreement with us in the formal traditional manner. Because Resina is the daughter in one of the major family lines of island chiefs, this procedure was essential to honor her ancestors, as well as the bloodlines and positions of the chiefs present with us. Further, this form of contractual agreement supersedes written paper documents which "come and go" along with various governments and administrations. So, if one wants to really seal a deal, these spirit-based contracts come first, followed by written legal documents for the lawyers and courts.

As we all sat is respectful silence, the Mata ni Vanua knelt down on the woven palm frond pallets which covered the floor and pushed the Tabua forward with his hands. As protocol required, he stared only at the floor while approaching the chiefly council. I sat on the side remembering my history studies about the old days of cannibalism in Fiji. Only just over a century ago, we, the bearer of requests and gifts could have been thrown into the cannibals' boiling pot if the tooth were rejected. Although we were in the 21st century, I said a little prayer that the tooth be accepted! It was!

We celebrated with what turned into an evening of an "a cappella" gospel singing and prayers. Out of respect for the deep, sincere Christian traditions of the villages on Kadavu, I asked if I could sing a prayer of thanks. My intention was to share this little prayer blessing as a gift and an indication of the respectful love with which we intended to exercise and maintain their traditions during our harvest contracts. As I finished, thinking that would be the end of the ceremony, a much greater blessing arose to touch our hearts. Suddenly, from the women's section in the rear of the longhouse, a beautiful soprano voice sang out a crystal clear note. It was followed by individual alto, tenor, baritone, and bass voices. The entire village responded vocally and built a gorgeous, sonorous, harmonious chord which energized us all and seemed to penetrate the now darkened skies outside the longhouse.

As it turns out, unbeknownst to us, this village had just won first prize in the inter-island gospel singing contest! The evening came alive with gospel "spirituals" from the island's two centuries of Christian tradition. When the evening was brought to a prayerful close, we emerged onto the village green. Looking up at the night sky, we were awestruck by the deep black velvet of the universe studded with billions of sparkling stars! It was as if the God of Heaven had cast endless jewels across the galaxy with ecstatic abandon. I hiked down the mountain trail to our boat on the bay in speechless joy.

So, as you can see from just a few of the experiences we have shared so far, our little project was carried forward not just by our strict adherence to solid science and government regulations in the United States. There has been a motivating set of signals from the forces of Nature and folks around the world touching the hearts and minds which has kept us on track. We have often wanted to give up when the going got tough. Just at those moments, I can hear the melodious sounds of the Kadavu village choir and take one more step forward.

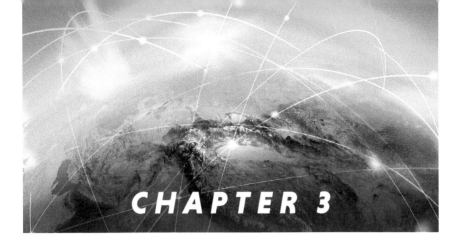

CHAPTER 3

DEVELOPING AND TESTING THE WORLD'S FIRST MANGROVE NUTRACEUTICAL PRODUCTS

Ted Anders, PhD

To ensure that we were creating safe, ethically developed, dietary supplements or "nutraceutical" products, we had to understand the phytochemistry of the red mangrove. Next, we needed to establish the first foundation stones of contemporary clinical observational data. Since we are the first in the "modern western" world to attempt developing a commercial nutraceutical derived from red mangrove, there just wasn't much data readily available. Because no one had analyzed red mangrove phytochemistry thoroughly for product development, I had to fund the initial laboratory studies in 2003, 2004, and 2005.

(Fascinating research is still continuing today, as we'll see in the next chapter.) The research was done with extra earnings from my global consulting practice, the investment assistance of William Elmhirst in Porlock, England, as well as investments from my parents Rev. Charles and Dr. Mary Anders, sister Rebecca Anders, and numerous patient friends and colleagues.

Here is a summary of the primary phytochemical activities we initially determined exist in red mangrove:*

- Anti-microbial (including compounds which are anti-viral, anti-fungal, and anti-bacterial)
- Anti-inflammatory
- Immune System Stimulating/Modulating
- Anti-pyretic (i.e. fever reducing)
- Anti-Oxidant

*Initial guidance on the most probable categories of phytochemistry to examine in the lab was provided by L. Caarl Robinson of Cedar Bear Naturales in Roosevelt, Utah. Caarl is a very well-informed herbalist and has been a consultant to Sen. Orrin Hatch of Utah as initial national botanical safety standards and ingredient guidelines were being developed for Utah and the United States.

These phytochemical functions are in direct alignment with the powerful reduction of colds/flu/Upper & Lower Respiratory tract infections reported in Fiji and which we observed in our initial test cases. Think about it. Colds are caused by rhinoviruses and require anti-viral (not anti-biotic activity) solutions. Remember, that was the primary treatment issue we had faced with my daughter, Natalie. Therefore, antibiotics prescribed for viral infections is not at all effective. Red mangrove contains several flavonoids which are

known to be anti-viral. Also, the rhinoviruses cause an immune system response which, among other reactions in the body, involves a histamine reaction experienced by the patient as swollen nasal and sinus tissues excreting mucus. These inflamed tissues require an anti-inflammatory action. Red mangrove provides the polyphenols which help reduce the inflammation.

Meanwhile, the immune system needs a boost in order to produce T cells to fight microbes. Red mangrove contains the polysaccharides which deliver this function. Further, colds which linger long enough to allow bacterial infections to take hold in the mucosal linings of the nose and sinuses, and then lower into the trachea and lungs, require anti-bacterial support. Red mangrove provides several compounds which are known to be anti-bacterial. When fever then emerges in an extended cold (or, initially, in a flu condition), something is needed to help reduce fever. Red mangrove provides a known anti-pyretic. Finally, to strengthen the body's overall immune function and sustain healthy cellular function, anti-oxidants are required. Red mangrove provides substantial anti-oxidant function.

The lab results clearly indicate the presence of active ingredients directly related to respiratory-related immune system infections. So, it was even more obvious to us we were on the right track in product development. What's more, each active compound we identified is known to be safe, natural and non-toxic to humans. In essence, red mangrove delivers the type of phytochemical compounds one would find in a carefully-designed concentrate of the healthiest vegetables and fruits.

Not only are the phytochemicals of its aerial rhisomes, bark and mature roots virtually non-toxic to us—through either ingestion or topical contact—it's own immune system phytochemistry seems to support ours in a rare manner; unlike any other single botanical of which I'm aware. I am willing to state, until, or if, I am informed otherwise, that red mangrove is one of the most ideal, healthy, life-form companions with us humans on the planet. That is no small claim. They deserve our close attention and protection.

The only ingredient which was called into question by emerging legal guidelines were small amounts of ephedrine alkaloids. Ephedrines were made illegal in the United States during the Bush administration due, primarily, to consumers' misuse of diet/weight loss pills which once contained them. Ephedrine alkaloids themselves, in natural plant concentrations consumed reasonably, are not harmful. In fact, they are quite beneficial and help ensure the rapid delivery of other helpful active ingredients to their designated sites in the body. The problem comes when a manufacturer makes products with high concentrations of ephedrines—or, more typically, the consumers who are desperate to lose weight think to themselves, "If one pill a day will cause me to lose 1 pound a week, I wonder what 5 pills a day will do?" In other words, it is not the ephedrine alkaloids which are dangerous. It is human, emotion-driven misuse of them which causes problems.

The federal court legal controversy which erupted between the Bush Administration (which insisted there would be absolutely no measureable presence of ephedrine alkaloids in products) and the position of the informed nutraceuticals/dietary supplement industry (which insisted there be a federal standard set for maximum content level of ephedrines in a product) ultimately was resolved in favor of the Bush administration. In any event, our forward momentum on product development and delivery was severely curtailed for two years while I investigated how to sustain reliable clinical effects for patients while ensuring our formulas had no measureable ephedrine alkaloid levels. Fortunately, as mentioned earlier, one of our shareholders, Dr. Nora Frey, is a Swiss citizen/ biochemist. She is very well networked into the community of pharmaceutical and food product development experts in Basel. As mentioned in Chapter 2, most pharmaceuticals are derived from plants. Therefore, the Swiss pharmaceutical and nutritional products community is replete with phytochemical specialists.

I flew to Switzerland and conducted meetings with these experts. As a result of the guidance I obtained, we were able to modify our formulation methods to eliminate measurable levels of ephedrine alkaloids in the final product; while still sustaining the dramatic, healthful, rapid response in the body. Needless to say, I felt like I had won a world series championship when we made it across this goal line!

Now that you have some perspective on the background lab research we did while developing and testing new respiratory and immune systems support products, join us now as we share with you the intriguing results of our first casual, uncontrolled client interview study and our first formal, "semi-controlled" clinical observation study. Remember, when we began our initiative in the late 90s and on into the first years of this century, there were very few studies reported, worldwide, on red mangrove phytochemistry in peer reviewed journal articles. There were *none* on red mangrove medicinal product applications. Dr. Amnon Levy of the United States Department of Agriculture and a well-known botanist and dietary supplement/food products researcher, conducted the initial global literature review for us. Based on the limited research available at the time, it was apparent our team was plowing new furrows in a relatively unknown field. Exciting!!

Dr. Ted Anders' Initial Client Interview Study

In 2004, I conducted a client interview study to establish the first contemporary insights into the efficacy of red mangrove extract products; in this case for colds/upper respiratory tract infections (URTIs). Subsequent to my study, Scott Carroll, M.D., co-founder of The Atlanta Allergy and Asthma Clinics, volunteered to conduct the world's first formal clinical observation study of red mangrove ingestible extracts in 2005.

Here is what I found after interviewing more than 75 clients, their representatives, (ages 2-80+) who had used "Fiji Tea" (today known as Respigard™).

Eight out of ten clients with reported "colds" recovered within two days (48 hours).

The reports for toddlers were made by their mothers. The majority of toddlers and older children were members of the Pinecrest Academy school community in Forsyth County, Georgia. The majority of the young adults and senior adults using the product were residents of greater metro-Atlanta, Georgia, Flagler County, Florida and Marin County, California. As I stated earlier, this information was gathered in interviews (in person or over the phone) and there had been no "controls" over the client's use of other cold/flu medications nor a monitoring of the timing of our product use in relation to symptom onset. The intention was to determine if we had created a relatively effective concentration of red mangrove—and to gather any reports of apparent "side effects" or a pattern of negative interactions with one or more standard over-the-counter (OTC) cold/flu products.

There were zero negative side effects reported; including in the interviews with those clients who used one or more OTC products.

Dr. Scott Carroll's Clinical Observation Study

When conducting research, it is essential to adhere to a conventional set of research practices. One of the most basic steps is to ensure there is no unethical or biased data gathering. Often, a scientist can be so heavily committed to "proving" a particular outcome, he or she can inadvertently (or, in the worst case, intentionally) misrepresent the data collected or report results affected by an unconscious bias. In strict adherence with good research practices, I invited Dr. Carroll, a widely respected pediatrician and immunologist practicing at The Atlanta Allergy and Asthma Centers, to conduct a semi-controlled study (as opposed to a full "double-blind" clinical trial which would have cost nearly a quarter of a million dollars, which I didn't happen to have available for this research purpose at the time.) Dr. Carroll had no economic connection with our companies nor would he obtain any gain dependent on study outcomes.

As background, a "double blind" study design is one in which neither the experimenter nor the study participant knows which product is being administered to a particular patient (i.e. the actual product or a placebo such as a neutral, inactive pill or a flavored liquid). Typically, such a study would also strive to control certain characteristics of the patient (e.g. age, sex, date of onset of a disease, etc.) and all primary variables in the patients' experience which could have an effect on the study outcome (e.g. use of other products while using the test product, hours of sleep per night, etc.)

Oftentimes, less controlled, but very informative studies are conducted as the initial, broad, learning curve of insights is being built up by a cadre of researchers in a new field of research or a new theoretical model. In our case, we chose the useful and affordable (because of Dr. Carroll's generous allocation of his time and clinic resources) "semi-controlled" model. The study did not select or group patients by age or sex or other demographic characteristics (with the exception of a subset of patients who were known to have recurring sinus infections annually—usually about the time of year the study was conducted).

Instead, Dr. Carroll conducted a straightforward, "common sense" study in which he tracked:

a.   the intensity of "cold" symptoms upon presentation in his office (ensuring, for study implication purposes, that the patient was presenting in the early onset phase of a "cold"/URTI);

b.   the basic demographics of the client (age, sex, clinical history of URTIs);

c. the use, if any, of OTCs or pharmaceuticals prior to and on the day of entering the study to receive the red mangrove extract;

d. compliance with the prescribed extract use protocol over the days following the patients' office visit

He observed 84 patients (ages toddler through 80s) and his results are reported in the following quote from Dr. Carroll:

"Over 79% of the patients who received the extract at the onset of their infection had complete resolution of their symptoms within 2 days. The common cold usually lasts 7-10 days."

Further, he observed no negative side effects or contra-indications with OTCs/pharmaceuticals. Dr. Carroll provided us with very important insights into the need to continue developing natural, safe, effective solutions. His views are very important and we are including them here in the form of the transcript from an educational program he conducted on our red mangrove extract we have previously called Fiji Tea, but now re-branded as Respigard™.

Transcript of Dr. Carroll's DVD Presentation

Hi, I'm Dr. Scott Carroll; I am going to spend the next few minutes with you talking about a remarkable product, Nature's Nurse, Respigard™, a completely natural and organic dietary supplement for treating and defeating colds and many of today's other respiratory challenges. I am the Senior Partner of the largest allergy and asthma clinic in the United States. I am board certified in two specialties: pediatrics and allergy asthma and immunology. As a practicing physician for over the last 36 years, I have become a strong proponent of a more natural approach to medicine. My overall goal is to place less emphasis on the pharmaceutical approach to treating patients and using natural alternatives that will often provide even better results and may have fewer, if any, side effects at all.

Think about this: healthcare is costing us 2 trillion dollars a year and the United States ranks a dismal 45th in the world for life expectancy. As much as one third of the expenditures do nothing to improve health, thanks to unnecessary treatments and tests. Even though medications can be life-saving, many are significantly over prescribed and often result in sick people becoming sicker, or dying. Even when drugs are prescribed correctly, over 100K people a year die from side effects alone. **It has become the 4th leading cause of death in this country.**

It is interesting to note that in the media drug ads, especially television, nearly ½ of the commercial is devoted to possible side effects. I think that as a society it would be wise to change our reliance solely on treating symptoms with pharmaceuticals. To me it makes more sense to treat the underlying causes of the problem, rather than just treating the symptoms. Many of our healthcare costs can be reduced significantly by making better choices concerning diet, exercise and the use of more natural supplements as a means to prevent disease and to maintain one's health.

This brings me to Nature's Nurse, Respigard™. I met Ted Anders, cofounder of Nature's Nurse, in 2003 at a seminar he was conducting promoting Respigard™. I kept an open mind as I listened to this man reflect back on his search for a treatment for his youngest daughter, Natalie, who was experiencing repetitive nasal, sinus and ear infections that just weren't responding to traditional pharmaceutical medicines.

A search that ultimately lead him to the Fijian island and Nature's Nurse cofounder and native Fijian, Resina Koroi, whose family harvests the exclusive extract of the Fijian red mangrove called Titi, which has been used for centuries to help the body's natural defenses fight colds and other respiratory challenges. Now, I had no idea if this stuff really worked, but I was at the very least intrigued. So, Ted and I had an affinity for each other right away. As I got to know him better, his knowledge and his integrity and all the wonderful people who are associated with Nature's Nurse Company and Respigard™, especially, Resina Koroi, I decided to conduct a study for him right away. I wanted to evaluate the clinical application of this natural extract. Now, as a side bar, let me mention this; doctors tend to prescribe antibiotics too often, especially in the treatment of upper respiratory infections, quite often at the insistence of the patients. They say, 'Dr., I need an antibiotic to get better.' Well, the problem is that over 80% of upper respiratory infections are caused by a virus and do not respond to antibiotics.

Antibiotics should be reserved for specific bacterial infections. So I conducted a study in my clinic with patients that had at least two or more of the common cold symptoms: runny nose, sore throat, cough, malaise, fever, headache.

Seventy-nine percent of my patients who received Respigard™ at the onset of their infection had complete resolution of their symptoms within 48 hours. This is phenomenal since the common cold usually lasts for 5-10 days. Pharmaceutical companies are allowed to launch new drugs based on only a 40-50% of improvement rate, so I was very impressed with the results of my study. In addition, I found that the immediate use, that is within 24 hours of the initial onset of symptoms, using Respigard™ many of my patients who had a history of repeated sinus infections experienced relief. And importantly, I did not record any side effects of

Respigard™ or any contraindications with other prescription pharmaceuticals, including blood pressure medicine, etc.

So, in conclusion, I really strongly encourage the listening audience to visit the Nature' Nurse web site at www.naturesnurse.com Learn more about the Nature' Nurse company, its cofounders, the product Respigard™, it's history, harvesting, overall benefits, indications, as well as testimonials from people just like you. Who would want to be without this natural organic supplement for defeating their family's colds in today's respiratory challenges?

Dr. Scott Carroll's DVD on Respigard™ is available on the Internet at: http://mediasuite.multicastmedia.com/player.php?p=qv99wyqt.

The entire article by Dr. Carroll, as published online by Nature's Nurse International, Inc., is included as Appendix A.

Continued Product Development and Physician Adoption

By 2008, we had gained substantial confidence in the safe, reliable efficacy of our red mangrove extracts. We had even gone so far as to develop an entire set of products built solely on red mangrove phytochemistry, or in the case of three products, blended with complementary botanicals selected to enhance certain mangrove phytochemical properties. In the case of each product, the reported client experiences were as reliably positive as those for colds/flu/respiratory tract infections. The entire line of products delivered an observable, positive result for the majority of clients in a matter of minutes or hours. **Due to our client feedback obtained through the sale of more than 10,000 test units of extract, we knew the world needed to know about red mangrove–based nutraceuticals.**

With the advice and assistance of one of our leading shareholders, Evelyn Hatzigeorgiou, in New York City, we decided to rename the main cold/flu product so that its very name indicated the power and function of the extract. After some deliberation and creative brainstorming sessions, we settled on Respigard™. With Evelyn's encouragement, we donated Respigard™ to a medical charity group in NYC. The charity was headed by Dr. Richard Brown, an integrative psychiatrist from Upstate New York. Dr. Brown's purpose was to assist 9/11 First Responder survivors with their severe respiratory problems resulting from having breathed in waves of toxic, microscopic particles of concrete, steel, asbestos, carpet, plastics, human remains, and an endless number of chemicals emitted from the burning, collapsing World Trade Center towers.

The feedback from Dr. Brown regarding patient response to Respigard™ was so positive our team was moved to tears as we heard reports of 9/11 survivors whose breathing was improving noticeably! An especially touching case is that of a National Guard leader, whose squad was first on "the pile" of the trade center remains. He told us he knew within a couple of hours at ground zero something was terribly wrong with the air. He began to have an extensive, repetitive nose bleed. However, as did thousands of other courageous first responders, he stayed on duty diligently seeking survivors in the ruins.

Seven years after 9/11, the leader's lungs were burdened by scar tissue, various tumors and chronic bronchitis. As we walked down the street with him in Manhattan, it was clearly physically painful for him—and emotionally painful for us—to hear his rattling, wheezing breathing. We suggested that he begin a daily regimen of Respigard™ to help alleviate the bronchitis. He did so and called to tell us his breathing was substantially eased within days. Of course we were thrilled for him. However, three weeks later we received an even more interesting update.

His specialists at New York Presbyterian Hospital had been monitoring the various cysts, tumors and scar tissue inside his lungs for several years. On a regular basis, they inserted a scope into the bronchial tubes to do a visual examination. To their surprise, some of his scar tissue was revising itself since the last exam. Apparently, according to his report, this just doesn't typically occur. His physician asked him if he had been doing anything differently or "off protocol." Sheepishly, he informed the doctor that he had been taking a natural product along with his prescription pharmaceuticals. He held up a bottle of Respigard™ and explained that he had been adding it to his nebulizer and inhaling the mist. (This was news to us, as well.) His physician encouraged him to continue and he did so for quite some time.

The stories of folks like this made an impression on physicians in the greater Manhattan area. We continued to communicate with and educate physicians and pharmacists in the region and received continuous, positive reports beyond the scope of our original focus on colds/URTIs. We received physician calls informing us that pediatric asthma patients were experiencing a gentle relief in their bronchial tubes and could sleep easier at night. Senior patients with emphysema/COPD were reporting ease of breathing and more energy. So much so that their daily use prompted several to contact us and ask if we could produce and sell a larger bottle of Respigard™ which would serve them on a monthly basis. We did so. The calls from folks in other parts of the country and in other countries who had ordered online were nearly uniform in their satisfaction with respiratory system relief. Of course, one botanical and one product resource can't resolve 100% of respiratory cases, but the red mangrove extract was providing relief for well over 70% of the client's challenges.

As alluded to earlier, there have been difficult times over the years when the going was rough to keep financing the companies. Simultaneously, we had to continue our phytochemical and product refinement research while continuing to pay our Fijian villages for our harvests and contract rights. We were expected to—and did—provide philanthropic support to impoverished villages in Fiji while educating government leaders on this important resource and our sustainable agribusiness methods. So many times, we wanted to give up in despair of the lonely road forward. Yet, we remembered those calls from clients. **One woman and her daughter called from New York City to say, "Please keep making Respigard™. We can finally breathe!" It is messages like this which prompted the title of this book, _Breath of Life._**

Broadening the Research Data Base and Sharing Red Mangrove Extracts Around the World

As I mentioned at the outset of Chapter 2, my main professional activity for the past 30 years has been as a comprehensive organizational development consultant on five continents. A project near and dear to the hearts of my team and me was the intensive Tibetan Children's Education project we conducted at the behest of a leading Nobel Peace Laureate. Our team includes some of the world's leaders in education reform through upgrades in administrative methods, instructional "best practices," alternative student and teacher evaluation, teacher development, and curriculum design. In early 2009, our team was invited by the founder of Tibetan Children's Villages (TCV) in India to provide a broad set of consulting services to the Tibetan school system for refugee students. The students live in Tibetan enclaves throughout India (many in very remote and impoverished areas near the India/Nepal/Tibet border areas). They are offered the opportunity to board, live and be educated in a Tibetan environment to sustain culture and language. (The school system is headquartered in Dharamsala, India.)

The school system leaders have had a primary objective to transform the school system known as Tibetan Children's Villages (TCV) into a system which can produce the world's top professionals and specialists. Their leader said, "You tell us what to do and that's exactly what we'll do." Sure enough, the entire system of administrators and teachers followed this call, came to our trainings, and added heartfelt passion and energy to learning a new educational paradigm and to changing behaviors and attitudes rapidly. My colleague, Dr. Charles Martin, head of The Center for Education Program Development and Evaluation at Georgia College and State University, sponsored much of the service project. They also monitored the two-year intervention and stated that they had never seen such dedication and rapid behavioral transformation. The instructional methods sustain to this day. Now, how does all this relate to red mangrove extract research? Here's how.

I travelled to the refugee camp schools in the northern town of Ladakh; high up in the remote Himalayas. We also served the Tibetan university students in Delhi at their SOS hostel and we served in Dharamsala at the base of the Himalayas. One year, I arrived in Ladakh in late Spring as the seasons were shifting. I was a guest in the Nobel Laureate's northern "palace"—actually an ornate temple with simple living and meeting quarters attached. I noticed so many of the precious little two and three-year-olds in the Montessori classrooms were suffering from colds; as were many of the adult staff and students at the hostel in Delhi. And, in the midst of all his responsibilities, the head of the TCV system, Mr. Tsewang Yeshi, was attempting to maintain an unbelievably busy travel schedule, host foreign guests, and administer a continent-wide system while being knocked down with a severe cold. Well, by 2010, I always travelled with several bottles of Respigard™. So, Respigard™ to the rescue!

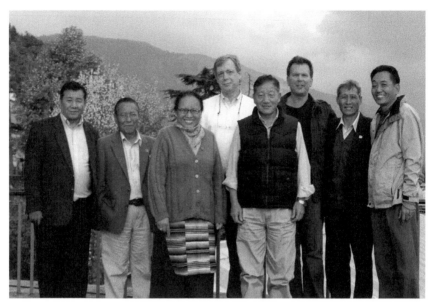

Dr Ted Anders with colleague Dr Charles Martin (to his right) and senior leaders of Tibetan Children's Villages (TCV).

We gave Mr. Yeshi a bottle at breakfast one morning in Delhi and we received a call that evening from one of his staff that he was much better! We contributed our extract to the family of the Manager/Dean of the Tibetan University student hostel in Delhi. Their bodies responded so readily they called and asked for more! We shared product with various teachers throughout the TCV system. Uniformly, they were very pleased with the rapid resolution of their colds/URTIs and were most grateful.

We also shared product and information with one of the leaders of an Indian university in Selakui who was assisting us at the TCV school adjacent to their property. Dr. Raj Trivedi is his name and he became a firm believer in our red mangrove extract after seeing its effects on students. He was so enthusiastic he offered to organize a clinical observation study for us in Delhi; where the vast majority of children—and a very large percentage of adults—suffer from repeated URTIs due to the extremely polluted air. (The air is so thick with visible particulate matter pollution most days that one could imagine scooping some up in a butterfly net.)

Raj was true to his word and organized a small trial with two leading Ear, Nose and Throat specialists in Delhi. One specialist practiced in a private clinic and one in a public hospital. Over the course of two weeks, the physicians included 15 patients in a study similar to the one conducted by Dr. Scott Carroll. The results are summarized in Table 3.0 below and concur with those found in Atlanta. More than 80% of the patients completely resolved (i.e. from severe, moderate or mild URTI symptom status to "normal") by the third treatment day and the remaining 20% completely resolved their URTIs by the fourth treatment day! These efficacy rates are almost unheard of among any type of health product; whether the product be a pharmaceutical, an OTC or a nutraceutical dietary supplement. Again, the plant showed itself to be a natural "Breath of Life."

Table 3.0 - Respigard™ Study in Delhi, India, 2011

	Patient Name	Treatment Days					
	Summary of patient VRTI sympton resolution with Respigard™						
		Day 0	Day 1	Day 2	Day 3	Day 4	Day 5
1	Mrs. Mohr	Moderate	Mild	Mild	Normal	Normal	Normal
2	Mr. Swaroop Mohanty	Moderate	Moderate	Mild	Normal	Normal	Normal
3	Mrs. Rashike Mathur	Severe	Severe	Moderate	Mild	Mild	Normal
4	Mr. Dharmendar Singh Sachhan	Moderate	Mild	Normal	Normal	Normal	Normal
5	Mrs. Anuradha Mathur	Moderate	Mild	Normal	Normal	Normal	Normal
6	Miss. Dharna Sethi	Moderate	Mild	Normal	Normal	Normal	Normal
7	Mrs. Rachna Sethi	Mild	Mild	Normal	Normal	Normal	Normal
8	Mr. G P Kathuria	Mild	Normal	Normal	Normal	Normal	Normal
9	Mr. Saahil	Severe	Moderate	Mild	Mild	Normal	Normal
10	Mr. Mridul Kashav	Mild	Normal	Normal	Normal	Normal	Normal
11	Mr. Shailender ATRI	Moderate	Moderate	Mild	Mild	Normal	Normal
12	Mr. Kuldeep Malik	Moderate	Mild	Mild	Normal	Normal	Normal
13	Mr. Mohammad Asiam	Moderate	Mild	Normal	Normal	Normal	Normal
14	Mr. R. Austin	Severe	Moderate	Mild	Normal	Normal	Normal
15	Mrs. Kailash Malhotra	Moderate	Mild	Normal	Normal	Normal	Normal

In 2009, I also made a trip to Cape Town, South Africa, to meet with the staff of Archbishop Desmond Tutu with whom I had traveled as a consultant on Nobel Peace Laureate projects. Father Desmond and I had appeared on the same speaking platform three years earlier at a peace conference in Bali, Indonesia. At that time, Father Desmond experienced the power of our red mangrove extracts and requested we send some to South Africa as a natural treatment for the rampant respiratory infections which plague HIV positive citizens. The Archbishop and his organizations have been very active in providing testing and support services to HIV patients in South Africa.

Imagine the healing which will occur around the world when our message of the power, safety and reliability of red mangrove extracts is shared globally.

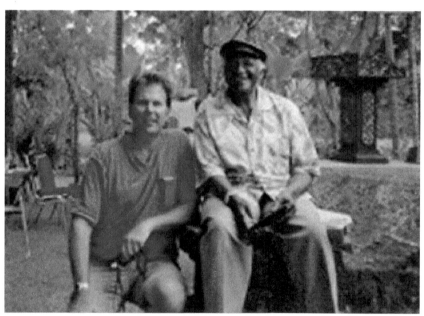

Ted Anders with Archbishop Tutu in Bali, Indonesia.

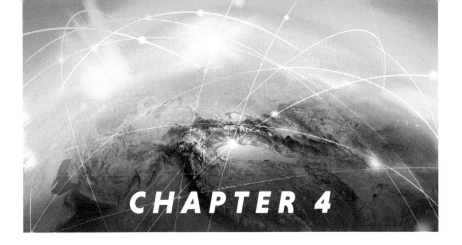

CHAPTER 4

WE'RE ONTO
SOMETHING AMAZING...
THE "MOTHER" OF ALL
NUTRACEUTICALS!

Ted Anders, PhD

UP TO THE PUBLICATION DATE OF THIS book, tens of thousands of units of Respigard™ extract have been produced and consumed by clients in the US, UK, China, Australia, New Zealand, Canada, and India. Over the years of our research and development project, global interest in red mangrove began to increase. While there was a dearth of information on red mangrove phytochemical function when we first re-introduced it to the modern world of nutraceuticals, there is now a growing awareness and interest within international scientific circles. Research is expanding. A partial bibliography of some of the references related to red mangrove phytochemical components and their impact on respiratory and immune function is included as Appendix B. After assessing Respigard™, a very astute health practitioner in New York City labeled red mangrove as "the mother" of all nutraceuticals; based on its ancient nature (350,000,000 years old), its own incredibly resilient immune system, and its comprehensive set of phytochemicals known to support healthy human physiology.

Parallel to the development of Respigard™, we gained much greater understanding of many more properties of red mangrove rhizome extracts. For example, hundreds of units of our more recent product, Skingard™ have been sold and clients repeatedly buy it in multiple quantities. Skingard™ is a special extract of red mangrove in which we enhance the concentration of certain polyphenolic acids shown in recent peer–reviewed research articles to enhance the rate of skin and capillary re-growth following damage to the epithelial layers.

Aqueous extracts of red mangrove have been shown to heal post-surgical wounds 50% faster than they would with standard wound treatments. In addition, when used topically, the extracts suppress microbial infection in an anti-septic function. The extracts also heal Herpes 1 and 2 lesion outbreaks very rapidly. Our clients report rapid healing of acne outbreaks, as well as rapid healing of cuts and abrasions. A research bibliography for each of these functional claims is included as Appendix C.

As I stated earlier, we have developed an entire line of products based on red mangrove phytochemistry and each one appears to be yielding similar rapid, reliable symptom resolution. For example, the Jointgard™ kit includes a topical salve and an ingestible liquid to be used in combination. These products build on the anti-inflammatory nature of red mangrove, as well as other characteristics. Focus group members report rapid relief which is sustained for 10-12 hours; with no noted negative side effects. In short, just considering the three products mentioned, there is so much promise from red mangrove research for human health and wellness! And the research is still in its infancy.

One can only be excited by the insights which will arise over the next few years.

Let's dig deeper into some of the basics we know about the phytochemical nature of red mangrove. Much is now known and we'll review several key points in this chapter. However, there are also some very interesting hypotheses being tested to determine why red mangrove is such a powerful, reliable support for human health. We'll present a few of those hypotheses with the help of Dr. Joe Ann McCoy, director of the Germplasm Institute at the North Carolina Arboretum in Asheville. She assisted us with the phytochemical functional analysis which we summarized in a matrix table which lists some of its interesting constituents, their function in our bodies, and numerical research references associated with Appendix B. See Table 4.0, below.

Target Phytochemical Constituents of Rhizophora mangle, L. red mangrove	Function — Anti-Microbial			Function — Anti-Inflammatory	Function — Anti-oxidant	Function — Anti-pyretic Analgesic	Function — Immune Modulation
	Anti-Viral	Anti-Bacterial	Anti-Fungal				
Quercitin	✓			✓	✓		✓
Umbelliferone (hydroxycoumarin)				✓		✓	
Luteolin	✓	✓	✓	✓	✓		✓
Kaempferol	✓	✓		✓	✓		
Isorhamnetin		✓			✓		
Apigenin				✓			✓
AHCC* - like Polysaccharides *red mangrove extract contains a very similar polysaccharide complex	✓						✓
Other Polysaccharides			✓	✓			✓
Salicylates						✓	
Other Polyphenols (including tannic acids)	✓	✓	✓				

Table 4.0

Key Phytochemical Constituents of Red Mangrove

Flavonoids (a sub-class of Polyphenols): Anti-Microbial, Anti-Inflammatory, Anti-Oxidant Compounds, Immune Stimulating

- Quercitin
- Umbelliferone (7-hydroxycoumarin)
- Luteolin

- Kaempferol
- Isorhamnetin
- Apigenin
- Catechin

These flavonoids are a sub-class of polyphenols which, individually or collectively, are anti-viral, anti-bacterial, or anti-fungal, while also providing anti-inflammatory, anti-oxidant, and immune stimulating functions in our bodies. Knowing the presence and function of these phytochemicals, it makes conceptual sense why our red mangrove extracts have such a profound effect on respiratory infections (which are caused by microbes, result in inflammation, and require anti-oxidant function and a strong immune response to resolve). Also, since topical wounds take longer to heal when they are inflamed and infected, the use of red mangrove extract directly on the wound area is, essentially, making a direct application of these anti-microbial/anti-inflammatory compounds into the wound site.

Of those listed above, Quercitin (a flavones) has been shown to be an active anti-viral (and anti-inflammatory, immune enhancing, anti-oxidant) in the human body. One study, included in Appendix B as item number 35, reports that busy working adults who took Quercitin supplements lost fewer work hours to upper respiratory tract infections than their cohorts who did not use Quercitin. Luteolin and Kaempferol have also been demonstrated to have anti-viral functions as well as anti-inflammatory and anti-oxidant effects. Luteolin also is known to enhance immune system function. Studies at the University of Ohio on lung infections are revealing that Apigenin is associated with the reduction of lung tissue inflammation caused in response to influenza. Meanwhile, Umbelliferone is known to have an analgesic (pain relieving) effect; which certainly complements the anti-inflammatory functions of the other flavonoids. After all, the pain we experience in our bodies is often due to inflamed tissues. So, all together, these flavonoids are providing a set of functions we need to recover from respiratory tract infections.

A representative research article and its summary abstract provide a deeper glimpse into the varied, useful function of red mangrove polyphenols. The research by Sanchez, et. al. is presented in summary form, below. The connection of this research insight and our Nature's Nurse products is made evident with the data presented in Table 4.1 which shows the presence of the flavonoid phytosterols referenced by the researchers in Cuba.

Polysaccharides (i.e. complex sugars): Immune System Modulating

• AHCC-like compound
• Other Polysaccharides

In recent years, studies of phytochemical action in humans are revealing that complex polysaccharides perform a critical role in the optimum performance of our immune systems. One well-known compound is called, Active Hexose Correlated Compound (AHCC) which is best known as a proprietary extract made from fungi; specifically, maitake and shitake mushrooms. We engaged Advanced Labs of Champagne, Illinois to assay the polysaccharides found in red mangrove. They reported the very substantial presence of a polysaccharide complex with molecular signatures very similar to AHCC. In fact, the polysaccharide was labeled by them as AHCC due to its close similarities. The most prevalent phytochemical constituents, by weight, in red mangrove rhizome samples are polysaccharides.

The fact that so much is known about AHCC due to its extensive use in standard, post-surgical hospital protocols in China and Japan (and as a dietary supplement in the United States), makes it possible to present some of the research on AHCC. Further, it will be a major insight for the nutraceutical-phytochemical science world when we (along with other researchers) clarify how the red mangrove is able to produce similar, powerful immune-enhancing compounds. Previously, it was thought compounds like AHCC had to be extracted in a proprietary manner and were known to be derived only from mushrooms (i.e. fungi). It was not thought they were produced readily by complex botanicals like mangroves.

Dr. Joe Ann McCoy of the Germplasm Institute in Asheville, North Carolina has been assisting us with the investigation into the source of the AHCC-like compound in red mangrove. Among many subject areas of expertise, she is an expert on endophytes; which are fungi living inside plants. She has provided brilliant insights into the endophytic "fungal factories" within red mangrove and challenged us with the hypothesis that endophytes could be the symbiotic "factory" inside the red mangrove plant which may be responsible for the presence of the immune supporting polysaccharides. Additional research is necessary to determine if this hypothesis can be supported. Such research is being conducted actively now in China, Saudi Arabia, and Caribbean/South American countries.

Salicylates: Anti-Pyretic (i.e. Anti-Fever) Compounds

Salicylates have been known widely as constituents that reduce fever. Perhaps the best known and most common is salicylic acid from willow bark. This acid is what we have all grown up with as "aspirin."

Umbelliferone, mentioned in the "Flavonoid" category, has also been reported as an anti-pyretic.

Note of interest: Research being conducted in India is focusing on the identification of constituents in mangrove which could be used as anti-plasmodials (which means anti-malarial) and the reduction of their fever-inducing action in humans.

Polyphenols (which include the Flavonoids, Phytosterols, Tannic Acids): Anti-Microbial, Anti-oxidant, Anti-Inflammatory, Epithelial and Endothelial Tissue Regeneration Support

This class of constituents has a wide range of functions in the human body. Polyphenols (as phenolics, flavonoids and tannic acids) are the most prevalent, clinically active constituents in red mangrove sample assays after the polysaccharides. Some are powerful antioxidants and can neutralize free radicals and reduce inflammation. Others slow the growth of tumors. Others have an anti-microbial effect. There are more than 4,000 polyphenols. We have not yet done an exhaustive assay of all that are contained in red mangrove. However, Appendix C includes a list of research articles which provide many examples of polyphenols in red mangrove which are responsible for the health functions just mentioned.

Polyphenol and phytosterol composition in an antibacterial extract from Rhizophora mangle L. bark.

Sánchez Perera LM, Varcalcel L, Escobar A, Noa M.

Department of Chemistry, Pharmacology and Toxicology; National Center of Agricultural Research, San José de Las Lajas, Havana, Cuba.

"Rhizophora mangle L. bark aqueous extract has antimicrobial, wound healing and antiulcerogenic properties. These properties could be associated with its chemical composition. To test this hypothesis, gravimetric, colorimetric, gas chromatography techniques were used to determine the preliminary chemical composition of this extract. Sephadex LH-20 Exclusion Chromatography was used by the fractionation of total extract and fractionation of low molecular weight polyphenols by liquid/liquid extraction. High Performance Liquid Chromatography was used to perform the composition in this low molecular weight polyphenols fraction. The extract presented polyphenolic structures (54.78%) and other structural components (45.22%). Polymeric tannins were the major polyphenolic component (80%) and 20% were hydrolysable tannins. Epicatechin, catechin, chlorogenic acid, gallic acid and ellagic acid were monomeric structures determined in this extract. Phytosterols (0.0285%): stigmasterol, beta-sitosterol and campesterol were also present."

In further pursuit of an explanation as to how/why red mangrove extracts heal damaged tissue in the form of topical wounds, gastric ulcers and apthous mouth ulcers rapidly and reliably, we learned more about those which are known as "tannic acids." We also learned about the fascinating interaction between polysaccharides and certain tannic acids which work together to increase new skin cell and capillary growth. This information was obtained as we developed our Skingard™ product. Table 4.1 shows HPLC (High Pressure Liquid Chromatography) graphs of the presence of three tannic acids: Ellagic; Gallic; and Chlorogenic. Research has shown (see article number xx in Appendix C) these acids to be active in the red mangrove's unique tannic acid/polysaccharide interactive function which supports rapid tissue regeneration. (The table also shows the presence of two of the many flavonoids we have studied; Quercitin and Chatecin.)

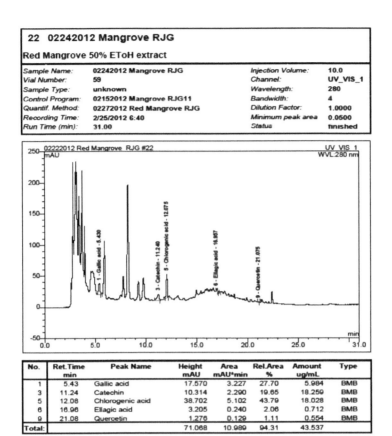

22   02242012 Mangrove RJG

Red Mangrove 50% EToH extract

Sample Name:	02242012 Mangrove RJG	Injection Volume:	10.0
Vial Number:	59	Channel:	UV_VIS_1
Sample Type:	unknown	Wavelength:	280
Control Program:	02152012 Mangrove RJG11	Bandwidth:	4
Quantif. Method:	02272012 Red Mangrove RJG	Dilution Factor:	1.0000
Recording Time:	2/25/2012 6:40	Minimum peak area	0.0500
Run Time (min):	31.00	Status	finished

No.	Ret.Time min	Peak Name	Height mAU	Area mAU*min	Rel.Area %	Amount ug/mL	Type
1	5.43	Gallic acid	17.570	3.227	27.70	5.984	BMB
3	11.24	Catechin	10.314	2.290	19.65	18.259	BMB
5	12.08	Chlorogenic acid	38.702	5.102	43.79	18.028	BMB
6	16.96	Ellagic acid	3.205	0.240	2.06	0.712	BMB
9	21.08	Quercetin	1.276	0.129	1.11	0.554	BMB
Total:			71.068	10.989	94.31	43.537	

Table 4.1 Sample Tannic Acid Flavenoid Profile

Red Mangrove Bark Bioactivity

Studies on extracts of red mangrove bark (which, of course, constitutes the outer surface of the rhisomes we harvest in Fiji) are now more prevalent in the phytochemical literature than when we began our project many years ago. The research supports the remarkable characteristics we have noted in our commercial products. Specifically, Articles 1-15 in Appendix C refer directly to the non-toxic nature (See Article 15) of red mangrove and its anti-microbial, tissue healing, anti-oxidant characteristics. Articles 1, 3, 4 and 9 focus directly on the wound and lesion healing supportive functions of red mangrove bark extracts. The article titles and research themes are provocative and promising. For example, Article 1 entitled, "Efficacy of *Rhizophora mangle* Aqueous Bark Extract in the Healing of Open Surgical Wounds," by O. Fernandez, et. al. presented in the journal, Fitoterapia, reports 50% more rapid healing of post-surgical wounds following the removal of piloidal cysts. And what's more, there were zero secondary infections noted in the entire treatment group of more than 30 patients.

Article 3, "Efficacy of *Rhizophora mangle* Aqueous Bark Extract (RMABE) in the Treatment of Apthous Ulcers: A Pilot Study," by E. de Armas, et al. and reported in Current Medical Research and Opinion, reports the rapid healing of apthous mouth ulcers using a rinse of red mangrove extract. Another example of research highlighting the tissue healing properties of phytochemicals in red mangrove is that done by P. Sanchez, et. al. and reported in the Journal of Herbal Pharmacology. Their article "Polyphenol and Phytosterol Composition in an Antibacterial Extract from Rhizophora mangle, L.", listed as number 4 in Appendix C, goes into great detail about the tannic acids (see Table 4.1, above) which seem to be involved in the rapid wound recovery noted with the use of red mangrove extracts. Article 15 includes a detailed report on a Dutch patent application in which red mangrove extract is an essential component in a medical device (skin patch) designed to heal Herpes 1 lesions rapidly.

The anti-microbial activity of red mangrove bark extracts is discussed at length in Articles 2, 5, 9 and 12. The anti-inflammatory function is discussed in articles 11 and 13. The anti-oxidant function is discussed in Articles 6 and 8.

The United States Department of Environmental Protection decision made in 1997 that red mangrove particulates are completely safe and non-toxic for topical exposure to humans of all ages is reported in Article 15.

Red Mangrove's Vital Role in Our Lives

Our contemporary world is just beginning to gain a more thorough insight into red mangrove phytochemistry and its powerful, reliable support of human physiological systems. As you can see from the cursory overview we've presented in this chapter, the promise for human health and well-being is significant. Let's close this review with one of the most exciting characteristics of red mangrove and give you an insight into just how significant it is. When you understand its unique nature, you can see the implications for its inclusion in a wide variety of medicinal applications; especially support of the human immune system. It also becomes glaringly obvious that we need to protect it!

Red mangroves are known to be "allelopathic" plants. In the case of red mangroves, this term means that the plant does not allow other botanicals to grow on, in, or around it. Some plants, bacteria, coral and fungi are known to be allelopathic. When you are walking deep into a mangrove swamp, you notice the only plants growing are mangroves! See our YouTube video entitled, "Nature's Nurse: Entering the Harvest" and notice as the camera pans the scene there is only mangrove present. Why? They don't allow other competitive or harmful botanical growth. Isn't this amazing? Not only is it amazing but it signals to the observer the presence of a very strong, protective immune system; with an additional ability to produce and excrete substances tailored to suppress competitive growth which could be harmful to mangrove survival. **After all, wouldn't mangroves have to contain the most reliable immune/protective systems to have survived as the oldest known living botanical species in its original form? Remember, they are 350,000,000 years old. They have been alive as long as sharks—and survived all the cataclysmic environmental changes which killed off the dinosaurs! These two species resist virtually all immune system threats nature (and man) throws at them.**

There are other life forms known to be allelopathic: rhododendron; eucalyptus trees; certain mushrooms and other fungi; and some coral and bacteria, to name a few. What's relevant to our appreciation of red mangrove is that most other botanicals which are allelopathic tend to be toxic to humans and/or animals. For example, when ingested at quantity, Rhododendron can cause respiratory failure. This reaction is the exact opposite of the impact red mangrove has on our respiratory systems.

Perhaps, now, you can appreciate why we stated earlier how rare it is to find a plant which is such a perfect companion to human life and well-being. In fact, I stated, it is perhaps the most companionable botanical life form to humans. It seems to help sustain balanced human physiology through support of our immune and other systems; when ingested and when used topically. **In short, it is vital to human health while also serving to sustain oceanshore and coastal ecosystems. Red mangrove is our partner in assuring human and planetary vitality!**

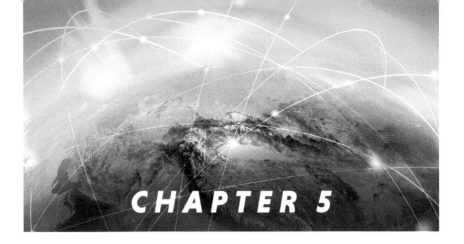

CHAPTER 5

THE NATURE'S NURSE ECO-SOCIAL BUSINESS MODEL

Resina Koroi

VILLAGE LIFE IN FIJI IS A COMMUNAL one where everything is shared and there is no individual property. To understand a little about how land is owned in Fiji I quote from the website of the Fijian Affairs Board website or iTaukei Trust Board who look after the vested interest of all iTaukei or the indigenous people of Fiji.

"Fijian or "iTaukei" land comprises 87 percent of all the land in Fiji and was permanently deeded by the British Crown in the 1880s, Put simply, it cannot be sold; it will remain forever as the property of the landowning unit unless it is sold back to the State and used solely for public purposes. iTaukei land is available for public use by lease agreements and leases can vary from 30 years for agricultural purposes up to 99 years for most other uses including residential, commercial and industrial leases."

The iTaukei owns native land in their collective groupings according to custom and tradition as follows:

- Land owned by titular heads of tribes e.g. Chief who for the time being holds the hereditary title of the "Na Ka Levu"
- Land owned by agnate descendants of a member of a tribe – Qele in Kawa
- Land owned by a Tokatoka (family unit). This ownership style is widely used in the province of Ba (where some of our harvest contracts are located)
- Land owned by the mataqali (clan)
- Land owned by the yavusa (tribe) and
- Land jointly owned by several yavusa.

Rights of the Landowners

The rights of owners of Fijian land over the parcels of iTaukei land allocated to the members are equal to the rights of owners of freeholders. These include the following to name a few important points:

- The right to occupy their land
- The right to use their own land for their maintenance or support
- The right to lease land to others and determine the terms and conditions of such leases acceptable to willing lessee
- The right of reversion, after the lease is determined at the end of its term.

With this in mind, our first step in establishing a business model that would benefit the villages and the business was to decide to deal directly with the villages, as they were the ones who would be affected the most. We had an environmental impact assessment done which was unheard of in those early days. We wanted to ensure that we would not be harming the environment or the mangroves in any way. My dream about my ancestors telling me that I was to be a good custodian of this magnificent plant kept coming up in my mind as we progressed through the years and has been a constant, gentle reminder that we have to protect and respect nature. Only then will the benefits of the mangroves be manifested fully.

The education of the villagers we dealt with initially about the importance of the mangroves in their villages was paramount. Ted led many sessions for villagers in the mangroves. At that time, we had some villages which had pig pens in the swamps and advice was shared that this was not a healthy practice because continued life of the mangrove depended on its being able to thrive in protected natural environments. Villagers were told about mangroves and the important part it played in their food chain.

Mangroves have a major role in the cultural and economic livelihoods of many villages along the coast in Fiji. Mangroves are known as the nursery of the seas and are the important foundation and start of a complicated food chain and are home to different types of fish and crustaceans. Mangrove swamps shelter young fish before they grow big enough for the reefs.

Mangrove forests are thus a food source for many coastal communities. They are a source of many Fijian herbal traditional medicines and act as sea walls and buffers protecting coastal communities from eroding under the force of ocean waves. They also act as natural filters of sediments washing off the land, thus keeping the reefs clean.

An extremely valuable but often overlooked function of the mangrove forests is their long term carbon sequestration capacity. As an important carbon sink, they suck carbon out of the atmosphere. The build-up of carbon-dioxide in the atmosphere contributes greatly to the thickening blanket of gases and global warming.

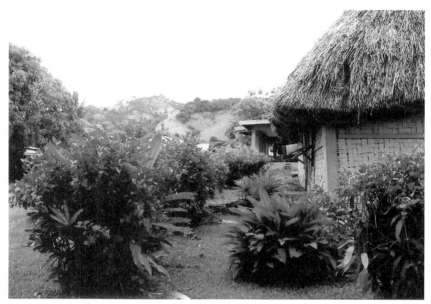

A traditional village home in Nadroga Province.

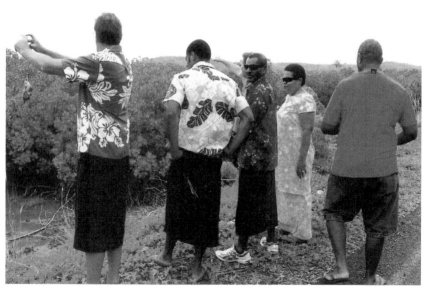

Planning for a new harvest zone prior to the meeting with villagers.

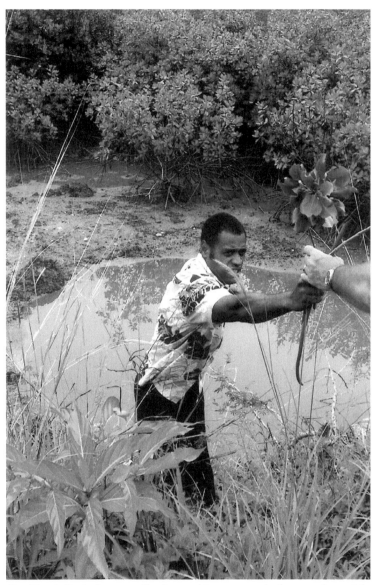

Benedict Koroi, Resina's son, collecting a rhizome sample from a planned harvest area.

Before starting a harvest, pre-consultative talks are held with village elders and then a time is made for us to address the rest of the villagers in a village meeting or the "bose va koro".

The villages we chose for the harvest were the ones that were self-reliant on the sea or on proceeds from their products sold in the nearby markets. Some of the land, as described earlier in this chapter as being leased out for tourism activities, were more well off and were not as reliant on their natural resources. We have not had any contracts with these villages.

At the village meetings, questions are answered and concerns addressed and some valid points have been raised for our consideration, such as the proper tools to be used during the harvest and the welfare of the women during the harvest. In some instances we have provided transport for all the village women to get closer to the mangrove forests without having to tramp through swamps.

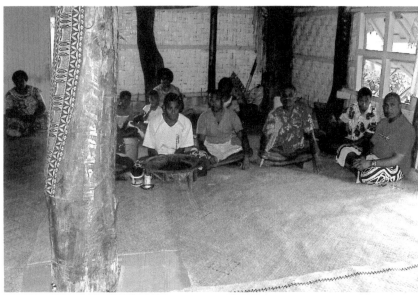

Harvest planning village meeting.

It is normally first decided before the harvest how many kilograms of Titi is to be collected in a manageable manner by the villages and the weight is divided equally amongst the villagers. The cutting of the Titi is done by women using machetes and shoulder bags for their harvest.

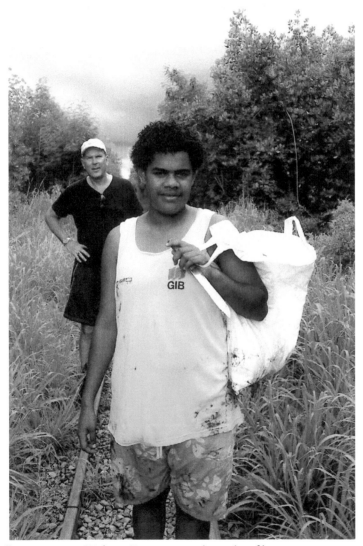

Tau village woman in Nadroga Province—in the midst of harvest.

Upon return to the village, the harvest of each woman (or man) is brought to the village meeting house and then inspected for accurate cuts and lengths. Each individual's harvest is then weighed publicly so the entire village knows how many kilos have been harvested and, thus, how much money is due to the harvester. The villagers know exactly how many dollars should be paid per kilo and how the funds are divided for the various tasks involved—and how much money goes to the village general fund. The entire process must be transparent and immediate to maintain trust and motivation.

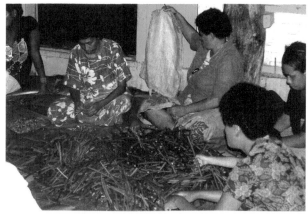

Women bringing their harvest into the meeting house.

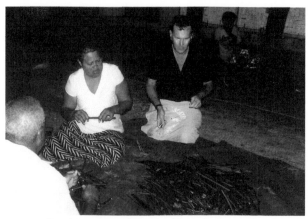

Resina and Ted (in required local village clothing called a "sulu") with the village leader inspecting the harvest.

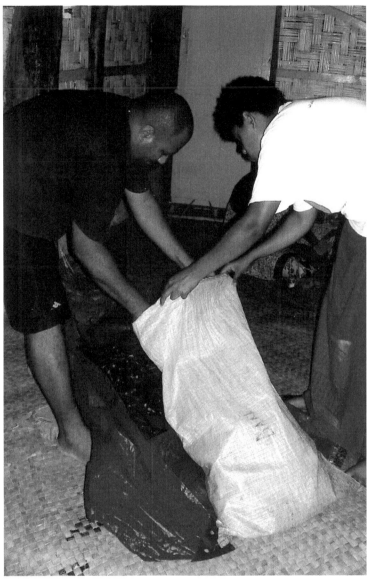

Preparing to weigh one woman's harvest.

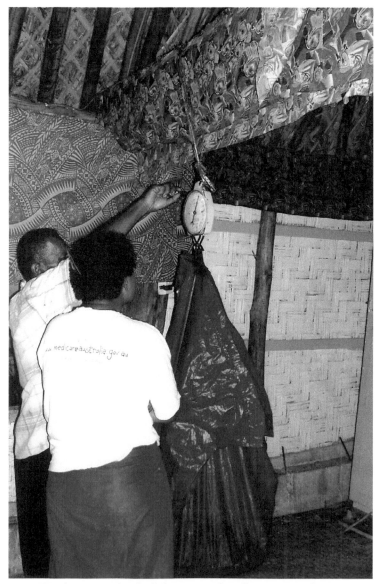

Weighing an individual's harvest in the village meeting house.

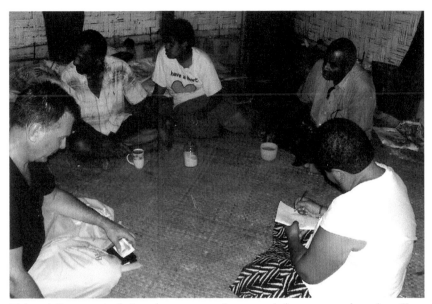

Ted and Resina calculating the payment due to each harvester and to the village general fund.

The cutting of the long rhizomes into small segments for pounding, to be done by local rugby teams, is generally done by the Village Women's Club to earn extra money for a project they have identified beforehand. Each village normally has a struggling rugby club eager to earn funds for their respective needs for local and national rugby matches and they are normally tasked to pound the Titi and dry it out to be packed again by the women before collection by our company.

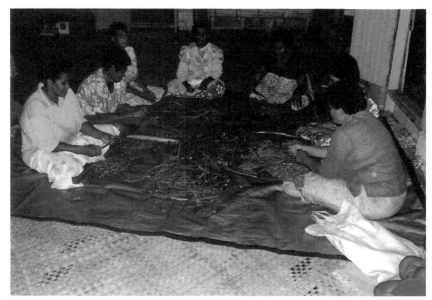

Women's Club members breaking the long rhisomes into smaller segments to fit easily into the mortar and pestle pounding tools used by the Rugby team members.

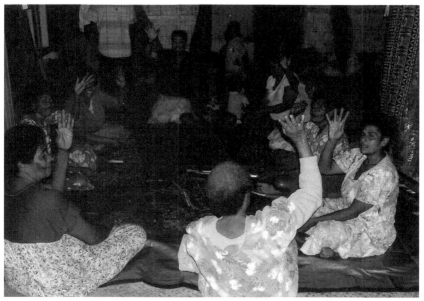

Another Women's Club waving to the readers of this book and users of red mangrove extracts around the world-sending wishes for good health to you!

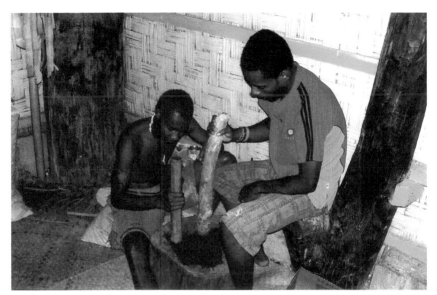

Rugby Team members pounding the red mangrove rhisomes into a mulch-like pulp which can be readily sun dried to a moisture level required by the USDA for importation.

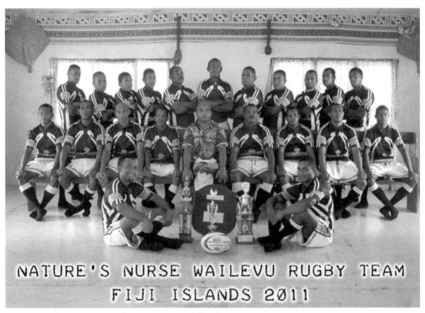

Proud rugby team members sponsored by the Nature's Nurse companies.

Throughout the years we have always stressed the importance of having everything done in the village so that villagers may earn the funds to be able to make their obligatory village and church contributions. This also enables them to sell their other products for the education needs of their children and daily family needs.

The whole harvest process itself is a lesson in humility, patience and deep understanding of the Fijian people; from the smallest child who runs up with a small amount of "Titi" to earn money for her grandmother who cannot make it to the mangroves to the tall strapping young man who wants to contribute to his mother's efforts to pay for schooling. Throughout the years we have gained insightful knowledge of the daily struggles of the grassroots people. Our Fijian and American team (which has become a multi-cultural "spirit family" and business partnership) is moved to help them thrive!

The carefully crafted methods we have designed are environmentally and culturally sustainable to ensure this new red mangrove nutraceuticals agribusiness we have created will serve the villagers' needs for centuries to come. Not only do the Fijians benefit. The health and wellness status of the whole world can now increase because of the red mangrove products created from the ancient wisdom and labor of the Fijian villagers with American scientific expertise. In fact, our red mangrove products have "gone global" via internet sales and due to their promotion on the Fiji national airline's duty free catalogue and carts on flights throughout the Asia Pacific region. The Fijian flight crews are so proud to bring traditional healing to the world on board trans-Pacific flights. Their enthusiastic smiles in the picture indicate how proud they are that a culturally sensitive, environmentally sustainable business model—which brings natural healing to all the people of the world—has its roots in their small, very special, pristine island nation.

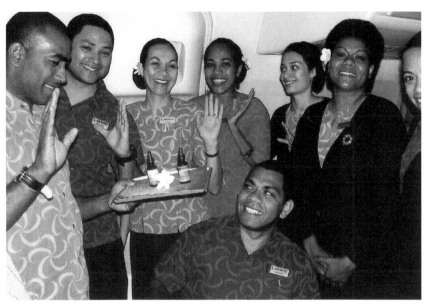

Fiji Airways In-Flight Crew selling our red mangrove product Respigard™ on board.

A Review of Poverty Concerns, Alleviation Goals and Sample Actions by the Fijian Villagers

While working in these villages, we kept hearing the good works the Minister for Women, Social Welfare and Poverty alleviation, Dr. Jiko Luveni, was doing for the needy and the women in these communities. We wanted to find out more about how our company could work together with her ministry. She informed us of the overall poverty situation and provided some important historical and global perspectives on poverty. Here is some of the important information she shared which has been written about her efforts.

Studies in Fiji found that income was unevenly distributed between different parts of the country and between rural and urban places, as expected. Fiji is no longer a country of self-employed, self- sufficient farmers, though the subsistence sector is an important source of livelihood. The study showed that various ways of calculating the poverty line gave a fairly consistent estimate of about 25% of households in Fiji living in poverty. However, many households seem to have incomes close to the poverty line.

The poor of Fiji are not necessarily the subsistence villagers, the unemployed, or the lazy. Most poor households have someone in paid employment, but the jobs they have do not pay enough to keep them out of poverty. Many households do not have access to land and sea resources, and even for those that do, subsistence does not provide a good livelihood.

Poverty pervades all communities, Fijian, Indo-Fijian, and others. The gap between the rich and the poor is increasing according to the Report. But much could be done to improve the situation with relatively little money, especially in housing.

Some Examples of Poverty Alleviation Projects

Earlier this year welfare recipients entered into business ventures with the help of the Ministry. The Government's strategy to provide welfare assistance with the purpose of empowering recipients is "bearing fruit" for certain individuals.

For 72-year-old Aborosio Marika Naleba of Waivola Settlement in Tailevu, Government's welfare assistance has allowed him to venture for the first time into the poultry business. Apart from poultry Mr. Naleba is now using manure from his poultry farm and started farming water melon, pineapple and root crops for micro commercial purposes.

"I would like to thank the government of the day for this amazing opportunity that has enabled me to improve the livelihood of my family. With the income earned I am able to even support the educational needs of my grandchildren as well. In particular I would like to thank our leader PM Bainimarama for initiating economic opportunities for less privileged people like me to build a good future by starting our own business.

"I would also like to thank the social welfare office in Nausori for their frequent visit to help me with my business. With this poultry project I am able to earn triple the amount of money which I used to receive as monthly welfare allowance. Now I am confidently living a much better life, using my time wisely and support my family without having to depend on anyone else. I like this project very much, even at this age I can work and provide for my family," Mr. Naleba added.

Empowering those under social welfare assistance to venture into workfare is one of the key strategies of the government which is aimed at alleviating poverty and promoting independent living. This is primarily achieved through the government's "Welfare Graduation Programme" administered by the Ministry of Social Welfare, Women and Poverty Alleviation.

The objective of the Welfare Graduation Programme, as reiterated by the Prime Minister Commodore Voreqe Bainimarama during the 2013 budget address, is to provide income generating and employment opportunities for the social welfare recipients.

"Fiji cannot support a culture of dependency. We must commit ourselves to the idea that poverty is a temporary state and as a society, we must uphold the value of work and self-sufficiency. When people move from welfare to work, they regain their self-esteem and confidence. Some participants in this programme have already set up their own businesses or are finding permanent employment. With an allocation of $500,000, the "Welfare Graduation Programme" focuses on moving the social welfare recipients from welfare to workfare," PM Bainimarama said.

Through the Welfare Graduation Programme, the Ministry works together with the National Centre for Small and Micro Enterprises Development (NCSMED), to assist the social welfare recipients to venture into economic projects.

The recipients are not only provided with the training, they are also assisted financially to start their income generating projects which is closely monitored by the Ministry. Last year the Ministry supported 32 livelihood projects with 39 sewing programs which are progressing well. Disadvantaged women around the country were given an opportunity to move away from poverty.

"The new partnership will create economic opportunities for women to venture into new business opportunities. This initiative will empower them with the necessary tools to become financially independent and improve their livelihoods and that of their families," Dr Luveni said.

One village spokeswoman said, "Our women's group has been in existence for the last 25 years and we do screen printing, sell jams and sweets to earn money. We don't have any permanent jobs and thus we have to depend on our husbands. We want to change this culture of dependency by becoming financially independent and now we have the plans to operate a wedding decoration business."

She said they can now start this business with the financial assistance from the Fiji Ministry of Women.

"We will organize social events and do decorations for weddings and religious functions in Navua. People can hire our services for price range of $50 to $100. We are grateful to the Ministry's financial assistance of $2000 and we have also been given a sewing machine to help us in this new project. The women can now utilize their skills to earn income for their families, we are so excited and looking forward for this initiative," she said.

Meanwhile, a separate women's group in Serua Province has also been presented with 20 sewing machines from the Ministry.

Wainadiro Women's Club president Mrs. Askilika Roseru said the new sewing machines have given them an incentive to pursue tailoring as a source of income generating.

Minister Luveni, while presenting the assistance to the Serua women's groups, reiterated that, "Empowering women will develop their income generating capabilities and add value to their roles into poverty alleviation and food security. Rural women are the heart of rural development and the ministry is maximising economic opportunities for these women to be agents of change in their families and communities."

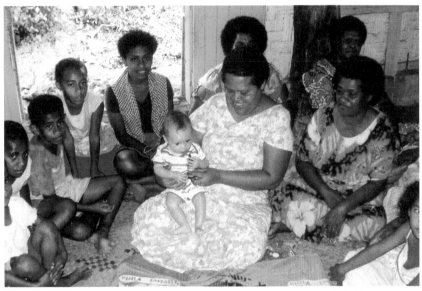

Resina holding her granddaughter, Eleanor, with village women and children. Resina gave Respigard™ to her 1 year-old granddaughter as a way to show the village women how their harvest had gone to the United States and been processed into a product for children. There was great pride among the women regarding their role in helping the world breathe through stronger respiratory and immune systems!

The Nature's Nurse Action and Vision to Alleviate Poverty in Fiji

With an active poverty alleviation initiative in place or being implemented in the villages, it made perfect sense that our companies, Nature's Nurse International, Inc. and Nature's Nurse Fiji, Ltd., join and complement the efforts of the government in trying to alleviate poverty in Fiji communities. We have been doing so by implementing our business model which re-educates the impoverished to sustain their environment for the future rather than using up resources for "a quick buck." Specifically, in the case of red mangrove, if a villager chops down the mangrove tree for lumber or firewood, he or she gets a one-time payment and the cash is soon gone—and the tree is gone forever. They lose the opportunity to participate in the permanent nutraceuticals economic sector we are creating. We are celebrating their nearly forgotten traditional harvest pruning practices and reminding them that if they will preserve their mangrove they can earn permanent annual incomes for their villages from sustainable medicinal botanical harvests. They can create a positive economic heritage for their own benefit, the benefit of their children, and the children of generations to come.

Indeed, a single harvest payment to one woman in a village—for just one day of her voluntary involvement in a harvest-- can exceed the typical monthly income of an entire impoverished family. Suddenly, it is possible for the family to save for the future, to repair homes, or open a micro-business of their own. Opportunities open for them—and this is what really alleviates endemic poverty!

Our greater vision is to assist Fiji with the creation of an entire new economic sector in agribusiness nutraceuticals. In so doing, we intend to help lift the nation's standard of living for the impoverished from third world status to a wise, balanced first world opportunity—within ten years of this book's publication. Through expansion of our sustainable harvests and employment in botanical extract production, we will enable communities to become self-sufficient. They will be able to take active ownership in the development of their own resources in an economically sustainable manner—all the while providing natural nutraceutical products from Nature's ancient wisdom to help heal illness across the world!

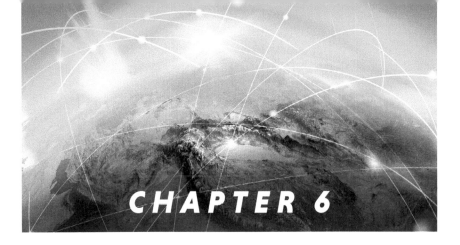

CHAPTER 6

CLIENT AND PHYSICIAN
TESTIMONIES

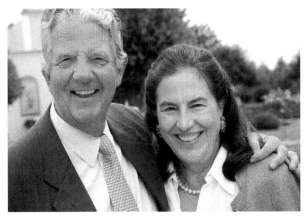

Prince Michael and Princess Christiana Von Habsburg.

"Dear Ted,
We fly a great deal and are always suffering from colds and respiratory infections. After taking your "magic drops" (Respigard™), we are no longer experiencing those infections! We will never again travel without Respigard™.
Thank you!"
Prince Michael and Princess Christiana Von Habsburg, Vienna and Budapest

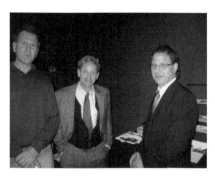

Ted, Dr. Mark Nessolson, and Dr. Benjamin Asher at an educational gathering at Slate Restaurant in Manhattan, New York.

Drs. Nessolson and Asher prefer to use natural solutions when possible and in the best interest of patient health and well-being. Here is what Dr. Nessolson said about our red mangrove extract following its successful use with his pediatric patients:

"Thank you so much, Ted, for providing this extraordinary product. I take it and I use it for my own family! Respigard™ is the product I recommend for coughs of any etiology."

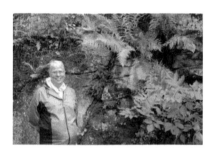

Client Kay Armstrong.

Kay Armstrong had this to say about her multi-year use of Respigard™ respiratory and immune system support:

"I've used Respigard™ for quite a number of years, and have become a proselytizer! If I ever have that scratchy throat or other symptom that says I might be coming down with something, I get started right away adding it to everything I drink! And normally I don't catch a cold. If one sneaks up on me, I get started, and it usually ends quickly.

I share bottles liberally with loved ones, particularly those who seem vulnerable to respiratory symptoms, and they all seem to do well with it, and ask for more!"

Kay Armstrong, Tybee Island, Georgia

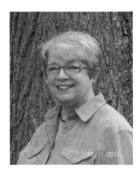

Client Jan Marriette.

Jan Mariette had this to say about her multi-year use of our red mangrove extract:

"I have personally used Respigard™ for a very long time (back when it was still called "Fiji Red Mangrove") and have always been awed by the way it immediately helps ward off or eliminate colds and upper respiratory issues. I've shared it with friends and family...and clients for a long time."

Jan Mariette, Reflexology, Inc., Savannah, GA

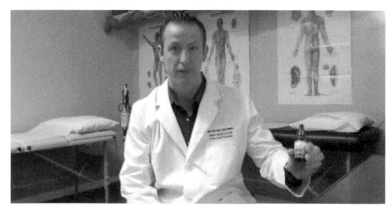

Dr. James McCall.

"Hi, James McCall here at Flagler Beach Natural Medicine. I am a licensed acupuncture physician and doctor of Oriental Medicine. I started using Respigard™ six months ago when I met Dr. Ted Anders. I was very impressed with the man, his integrity and his commitment to natural health. Since then, I've used it for patients who have asthma and I've seen some great benefits. I've also used it for cases of upper respiratory infections—including in pediatrics. We have seen great results and we highly recommend Respigard™ for our patients."

Dr. James McCall, Flagler Beach, Florida

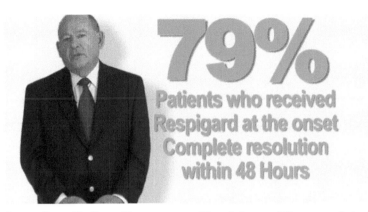

Dr. Scott Carroll, founding partner The Atlanta Allergy and Asthma Clinics, and Medical Advisor to Nature's Nurse Companies.

Dr. Carroll conducted a study on patients with Colds/Upper Respiratory Tract Infections in his Atlanta Allergy and Asthma Institute. Each patient presented with at least two of the typical symptoms of the common cold. After just 48 hours, 79% of patients exhibited complete resolution of the common cold—with no negative side effects reported.

Dr. Scott Carroll, Atlanta, Georgia

Pamela Soukup

"I have severe asthma and have been using Respigard™ for over five years. It has been very helpful in heading off respiratory illness, when I take it at the start of a cold. If I take it after the cold has taken hold, it will shorten the length of my illness. This has been very successful for me, so much so that now my husband, my daughter, my sister and her family (including grandchildren) are all using Respigard™!

Pamela Soukup, Sunnyside, New York

Beverly Fisher

"I am a semi-retired woman who is an educational and business consultant. I travel extensively and am exposed to a variety of microbes on aircraft and in schools. When I heard of Respigard™, I was hopeful I had found a travel companion that would boost my immune system and keep me healthy. My routine quickly became taking Respigard™ four days before traveling, everyday while on the trip and four days following my trip. I can honestly say that with Respigard™ I have stayed totally healthy while being exposed to those pesky travel germs.

Beverly Fisher, Tampa, Florida

Dr. David Jin

As a clinician-scientist in the areas of internal medicine, hematology, oncology and regenerative medicine, I have reviewed and studied many natural products over the years. Your Fijian red mangrove extract has always amazed me with the exceptional quality and excellent efficacy for helping patients with respiratory and pulmonary ailments. In my practice, I found your product particularly beneficial for patients with asthma, pneumonia, TB, COPD, and even with palliative effect in patients with lung cancer, muscular dystrophy and multiple sclerosis. Recently, I helped establish the E. J. Corey Institute of Biomedical Research (CIBR) in China (Professor Corey of Harvard University is the 1990 Nobel Prize Laureate in Chemistry), and I am the director for the center of excellence for translational medicine there. Ted, it has been our common vision and passion to initiate a public health campaign in China targeting respiratory and pulmonary health in light of the severe air pollution and smoking. Using CIBR as a platform, it will be quite a privilege to initiate such a campaign in China with you and your Respigard™ team."

David Jin, M.D., PhD, Staten Island, New York

Nicole McDaniel-Richards

"In my 22 years as a consulting herbalist I have never experienced an herbal product that works as quickly as Respigard™. Most of my clients tell me they feel relief from respiratory discomfort in less than 30 minutes after the first dose. I have used Respigard™ on my son when he had a fever. After dosing him every two hours for six hours, his fever broke. We have used red mangrove for poison ivy and canker sores with instant relief. My client with COPD tells me it helps him breathe better and my client who usually has eight asthma attacks a year says she has not had an attack since using Respigard™. It is the first thing I turn to for any respiratory and immune distress."

Nicole McDaniel-Richards, Holistic Herbalist, McDonough, Georgia

Sarah Ernest

"As an herbalist and naturopath with a passion for children's health, I'm always searching for natural options for my own children. I tried Respigard™ for the first time with my one-year-old daughter, who was presenting with a runny nose and sneezing. Fearing an allergy to Echinacea, I searched for an option that would help her symptoms as well as her immune system. Within two minutes of giving her the Respigard™ her nose stopped running and her sneezing stopped for several hours. The product tasted great so I didn't have to force her to take it, which was also a huge bonus."

Sarah Ernest, Covington, Georgia

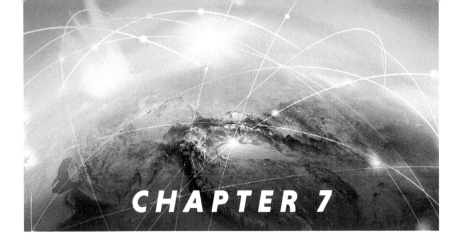

CHAPTER 7

THE FUTURE OF NATURAL MEDICINE COLLABORATION AND RESTORATION OF THE PLANET

George Briggs, Executive Director,
The North Carolina Arboretum
(An affiliate of The University of North Carolina)
Chair, Board of Directors, Bent Creek Institute, Inc.

(Opening and Closing Remarks by Dr. Ted Anders)

WE HAVE TAKEN A SLOW, PEACEFUL PATH to create products based on the healing properties of red mangrove. We have adhered to the highest ethics and standards.

We have been blessed to be noted for our efforts and invited by institutions of distinction to collaborate in a consortium of education, NGO, for-profit and government agencies. Yes, there must be profit and a profit motive in the economic systems of today. Yet, profit alone cannot be the only success criterion.

For our species to survive into the future with a planet that can sustain us, and itself, corporate success indicators must include measures of improvement within the ecological and human system "supply chains" from which profits are derived. And going forward, our species must learn to live more gently on the planet—and remember it was once a balanced, flourishing garden—which we have now virtually destroyed.

The evidence of our destruction is readily apparent: a radiated Pacific marine environment from the Fukashima Nuclear Reactor debacle; a poisoned Gulf of Mexico caused by the BP Deepwaer Horizon spill; and a thawing Arctic tundra now releasing more methane gas than all other sources combined. Thus, these events and others are warming the planet, melting the ice caps, raising ocean sea levels, destroying animal hunting grounds, and creating chemically toxic urban and suburban environments within which fetuses are struggling to be born and children are facing more neurological and related learning challenges than ever before in history.

In short, it is our responsibility as humans to restore "the garden" or neither we nor it will survive. Therefore, it is fitting that our red mangrove project has been nurtured within a garden research environment on the grounds of The North Carolina Arboretum which is affiliated with the University of North Carolina in Asheville. The following wisdom shared by its founder and Executive Director, George Briggs, are balanced words of wisdom for all of us. He presents a model of collaboration which nutraceutical corporations and supportive organizations can replicate worldwide.

George Briggs, Executive Director, North Carolina Arboretum:
Botanical gardens and arboreta, as public institutions designed to cultivate connections between people and plants, have long played key roles in human health, wellness and happiness. From their earliest history, when a primary purpose was to serve as the living "apothecary" of plants to be used in addressing health and wellness issues, these organizations have served as stewards, conservators and interpreters of the plant world.

In current times public gardens have broadened their mandates to include a wide variety of functions and regional roles. At their core, as plant collections, they exhibit plants that are native to a region, plants that are valued for their landscape function regardless of origin, or plants occupying various other ecological, botanical or functional categories. Thus, the plant collection is leveraged into education, research and demonstration purposes, and frequently targeted toward plant conservation. A public garden may work with plants located in their natural habitats (*in situ*) or in cultivation on site (*ex situ*).

The Search for Economic Relevance

As a past president of the American Public Gardens Association and the executive director of The North Carolina Arboretum, an affiliate campus of The University of North Carolina system that is located in the biologically-rich Southern Appalachian mountains of Western North Carolina, I have had the privilege of working within this context for many years. Rather than reacting to these monumental changes in society and the world of plants, The North Carolina Arboretum has targeted ways in which we can both celebrate our region – its beauty and its heritage – and provide leadership in advancing the role of an arboretum in 21st century ecological and environmental terms.

Central to this search has been attention to state and university system priorities and a thoughtful analysis of our regional uniqueness; and where these factors may provide a competitive advantage. If the Arboretum at its inception in the mid-1980's was to become a serious contributor to the economic and community development of our region, we had to identify key long-term tactics that would collectively support that strategy. First and foremost was an ironclad commitment to the institutional vision, mission and values that would collectively serve as our "north arrow" in guiding the way. Any commercial endeavors in the future would have to be aligned tightly with this commitment.

While we knew ourselves quite well as an Arboretum and the forces at play within our professional domain, we were not as familiar with the economic development community. Thus, we set about developing that familiarity by attending events and conferences, meeting economic development professionals, learning existing strategies and activities, and understanding funding mechanisms. Moving out of our professional comfort zone, we explored how the economic community might view an arboretum as a possible partner in their overall goals. Over time, the uncomfortable became familiar, and in time, the familiar became more comfortable.

The North Carolina Natural Products Association: Incorporated in 2001, this new organization brought together a widely diverse array of scientists, growers, manufacturers, retailers, government and university officials and others into a formal, organized, and collaborative network.

The Western North Carolina Biotechnology Advisory Committee: Established by the North Carolina Biotechnology Center, this board of regional and civic leaders focused on the economic development aspects of building the natural products sector. We served as the host site and chair during early development.

The North Carolina Arboretum Germplasm Repository: A scientific seed bank and extract collection of Southern Appalachian medicinal plants, and a central and highly reliable resource for research and product commercialization efforts, we believed that we would serve innovation best by providing a central source of easily accessible R&D materials.

The Bent Creek Institute, Inc. (BCI, Inc.): This independent nonprofit corporation, partnered with The North Carolina Arboretum by means of a broad Collaboration Agreement endorsed by the University of North Carolina (UNC) system, serves as the bridge between the Arboretum's research and germplasm collection and the commercial natural products market. The leader of BCI, Inc., Greg Cumberford, is a nationally noted industry expert and now consults and works with natural product companies worldwide.

The United States Botanical Safety Laboratory: Recognizing the problems associated with identity, contamination, adulteration and purity in the natural products industry, BCI, Inc., in partnership with UNC campus laboratories, Asheville-Buncombe Technical Community College and the North Carolina Community Colleges BioNetwork, a new North Carolina Research Campus, and other partners, created a new model for high quality, reliable product testing. By working together as a consortium, these labs receive blinded (anonymous) samples and produce test results that address plant identity, heavy metal, microbial, pesticide and other common forms of quality problems. The resulting data is unblinded and consolidated into a university-based, non-profit generated Certificate of Analysis that provides the client with reliable, unbiased third-party authentication.

Nature's Nurse: This inaugural "incubation" project represents the first fledgling company to be based at The North Carolina Arboretum as a case study and means of synergistically growing our mutual education and economic strategy. Based in the U.S. with business relationships in Fiji and predicated on the medicinal qualities of Fiji's Red Mangrove tree, Nature's Nurse represented a company that integrated our complex international, conservation and "natural biotechnology" focus as an institution, while also serving as a learning experience toward fostering local natural product entrepreneurs and companies.

The Broader Perspective

Our work and learning curve related to natural products have continued to expand over time. National concerns over health care cost escalation, the need for new therapies in battling disease states; greater personal responsibility for wellness through diet and exercise; adulteration and contamination problems in natural products and dietary supplements; antibiotic-resistant organisms, and other factors have become important in crafting a future vision for future health and wellness.

In addition to these human health concerns we continue to experience threats to global biodiversity due to loss of habitat, invasive exotic species, changes in weather and climate patterns, and other phenomena while we become increasingly capable and interested in drug discovery and new forms of therapy from bioactive compounds found in natural sources. Through advances in life sciences, we are now able to validate the efficacy of these bioactive components in ways that were unavailable to us just decades ago, thus making them much more available as legitimate as a component of a medical treatment plan.

All of these circumstances, following many decades of medical reliance on the single compound pharmaceutical model, are opening up new and innovative approaches to maintaining health and wellness. This movement toward greater personal health responsibility and prevention requires that we also take greater responsibility for the natural biological resources that will likely be the source of new discoveries and strategies for both preventing and treating diseases.

What Lies Ahead?

As represented by **Nature's Nurse**, strategies for natural product development now require an ever-increasing reliance on plant knowledge, sustainable practices, product formulation issues and a better understanding of both regional and international plant relationships. For example, many of our eastern North American plant species have counterpart species in Asia, known as disjunct or vicarious species.

If a particular plant has been used for thousands of years in Traditional Chinese Medicine, for example, might its botanical cousins elsewhere be a good place to explore for other beneficial compounds? (Note from Dr. Anders: In fact, the red mangrove (*Rhizophora mangle, L*) which Nature's Nurse harvests in Fiji is the same genus and species as that found in Florida, Cuba, Mexico, and Latin America (collectively known in the US Herbs of Commerce as "American Red Mangrove"), yet the unique varietals which have hybridized in Fiji may have strengthened the phytochemistry and its relevance to human wellness. This comparative research opportunity is on the list of future collaborative initiatives.)

It is also likely that future research efforts will continue to focus on endophytic fungi, organisms that live beneficially within plants and which may express the same traits as the plant compounds themselves. These organisms function in plants similar to the gut flora in humans, synergistically assisting in digestive and other biochemical processes in the body. This approach of isolating and cultivating endophytic fungi, if successful for certain forms of endophytes, would provide potential avenues of product manufacture that could bypass traditional agricultural processes. **In fact, Dr. Anders, in collaboration with Dr. Joe Ann McCoy of the Germplasm Institute and Greg Cumberford of Bent Creek Institute, are culturing and investigating the hypothesis that the powerful polysaccharide compound in red mangrove provides an immunomodulating function in the human body which is very** similar to that of **Active Hexose Correlated Compound;** which is a proprietary extract previously only available from certain mushrooms.

The interesting challenge in all of this is that while globally-based genetic research and plant sharing is a beneficial factor in drug and product discovery and advancement, it is of concern from the invasive exotic species perspective in such diverse issues as human, ecological and civic health. And, from an economic and commercialism perspective, what motivates a company, or a country for that matter, to work with natural materials or products that are more difficult to protect with patents or other forms of intellectual property.

Therein lies the wisdom in the **Nature's Nurse model.** Rather than exploiting a natural resource of Fiji by simply harvesting and shipping, this model represents a collaborative international model of business: sustainable harvest methods that employ citizens of Fiji; joint efforts at building a reliable and pure supply chain; contributions by **The North Carolina Arboretum Germplasm Repository** and the **Bent Creek Institute** to facilitate product formulation and identity validation services; partnerships with granting agencies and existing business, health and manufacturing interests; and numerous other partners to create a viable and contributing end product. Unlike many companies and products with disparate, disconnected and frequently unaccountable elements from field to shelf, **Nature's Nurse** represents a holistic approach to value creation where each party to the process not only contributes to the overall quality of the final product, but shares in both the investment and the returns in crafting an innovative, sustainable model with products that are free of adulterants, contamination and adverse exploitation of either people or environment.

All of this leads to the conclusion that Nature's Nurse is a fitting company as an initial incubation model for The North Carolina Arboretum and its associated partnering organizations. The Arbo-

retum strives not only to spawn a new natural products industry sector for the Western North Carolina region, but also to address national and global wellness and challenges while maintaining an eye toward economic, environmental and social value at every level of corporate activity. Nature's Nurse company, from its inception, has been graced with well-educated and process-oriented leadership that coordinates well with the mission of The North Carolina Arboretum and the Bent Creek Institute.

Conclusion

Unlike most new entrepreneurial endeavors that focus on developing a new product or technology, a company like **Nature's Nurse** has a far more comprehensive challenge in getting to manufacturing and market. Of course, all of the basic steps would apply, such as proving the concept, creating the brand, determining manufacturing protocols, designing packaging and undertaking distribution and sales.

In the case of **Nature's Nurse**, the key ingredient and the key management and harvesting relationships are half a globe away from the U.S. market. The heritage of use is interwoven into the history and ecology of Fiji, as is the empirical evidence of efficacy. Understanding the growth characteristics of red mangrove in order to protect both the ecological health and the company's supply chain is essential. As a natural product to be ingested, there are research requirements and standards, as well as protections that are more stringent than many other types of products headed to market are required to navigate.

The public-private partnership created by **The North Carolina Arboretum**, **The Bent Creek Institute, Inc.**, and **Nature's Nurse** represents an important new means of economic development by means of orchestrating a highly diverse and global culture of interests behind a single idea. None of these partners can afford to rely on previous models for success that are now woefully out-of-date — reliance on single sources of revenue and expertise, inordinate control over all phases of operation, absence of cross-functional collaboration and transparency, exploitation of supply sources, and inadequate attention to quality standards.

Rather than solely a company, **Nature's Nurse**, for **The North Carolina Arboretum** and **The Bent Creek Institute**, represents an innovative relational step into the future. Within these relationships lie a refreshing business model built on trust, accountability and honesty – all with an exceedingly wide geographic reach.

If we are successful in building a profitable triple bottom line for the three partners, we will all be even more inspired by the accompanying beneficial effects on human, ecological and economic health worldwide.

George Briggs

Looking Ahead...

We humans have reached the point in history at which it is essential we awaken to the truth that we are not separate from the Earth. Our bodies are "of it." Our hearts beat because of Her electromagnetic fields. We breathe because She breathes. If She loses her vitality, we die. It is that simple. As a species, we have completely lost our way in relation to our physical and Spiritual roots. Our families and friends who have helped bring red mangrove forward from the mists of time into your homes and clinics make this simple request: Love and respect one another and the living organism we call Earth, in every instance, at every key decision point in life. If we do so, our descendants and our Host, Earth, will thrive. If not, we will become another example of destruction and extinction. Surely, with the powerful pathways of Faith adhered to by the vast majority of human inhabitants, we can find a new Common Ethic which assures the survival of All.

Ted Anders, PhD

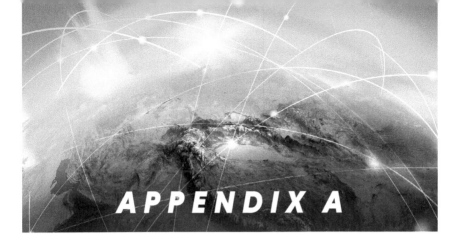

APPENDIX A

FULL TEXT OF DR. SCOTT CARROLL'S RED MANGROVE EXTRACT STUDY ON COLDS

The Effect of Fijian Rhizophora Mangle
(Red Mangrove) on The Common Cold

Scott Carroll, M.D.
December 2005

ABSTRACT

Background

THE FIJIAN SOCIETY HAS USED RHIZOPHORA MANGLE for over 100 years as the primary traditional treatment for the common cold and related symptoms. The aerial rhizomes of Rhizophora Selala, Rhizophora Stylosa and Rhizophora Samoensis were recommended to the Nature's Nurse, Inc. research team by village herbalists and members of the Biology Department at University of the South Pacific as being the most effective remedy for rapid elimination of head and chest congestion, runny noses, and other typical symptoms of a common cold.

Methods

A combination of research methods incorporating anthropological, ecological, behavioral and botanical field methods, along with laboratory analysis of the traditional herbal decoction of Rhizophora, were conducted over a five year period from 1998 - 2003. On the basis of this research, it was determined that a water-based decoction or a specific type glycerin-based fluidextract (100% alcohol-free) of a blend of the Fijian aerial rhizomes into a concentrated fluidextract are effective. In this study, clinical self-reports were obtained from 84 individuals using a standardized clinical report form and interview to collect protocol compliance and product efficacy data. The product tested is known as Fiji Titi /Fiji Tea.

Results

Seventy-nine percent (79%) of patients experienced substantial to complete relief of cold-related symptoms within 12-48 hours of initiating the recommended usage protocol.

Conclusions

The basic hypothesis of this observational study was: a water-based decoction or specific glycerin-based fluidextract (100% alcohol-free) of Fijian Rhizophora mangle delivered via a fluid extract concentrate would produce a rapid (12-48 hours), significant-to-complete reduction of cold-related symptoms in patients experiencing symptoms of the common cold. The hypothesis appears to have been supported. The results warrant further controlled, comprehensive clinical trials.

INTRODUCTION

The purpose of this observational, clinical report study was to monitor the impact of Fijian Rhizophora mangle on the common cold and related conditions. A general literature review on the traditional medicinal uses of Rhizophora mangle worldwide yielded general insights into the possible medicinal effects of Rhizophora mangle. A member of the Nature's Nurse, Inc. research team, Amnon Levi, PhD. produced a summary of the available literature; a subset of which is included as Appendix A. However, the literature review yielded minimal insights into the uses and efficacy of Fijian Rhizophora. Thus, the primary data source was the reports of herbal traditionalists in Fiji who were familiar with the historic anti-microbial uses and impact on the common cold and related symptoms. Their reports were corroborated by the Chief Pharmacist in The Fijian Ministry of Health. His letter indicating the recognized, safe use of Fijian Rhizophora is included as Appendix B. Additional safety evidence was obtained when product research and development revealed Rhizophora mangle to be recognized by the United States Department of Agriculture as an approved dietary supplement. Rhizophora mangle is listed in the directory, "U.S. Herbs of Commerce" as an approved dietary supplement. Additionally, our constituent analysis at Terradyne Labs of the raw rhizome supported the proposition that the plant is safe for human consumption.

The Fijian society has used the aerial rhizomes of Rhizophora mangle (Stylosa, Selala and Samonensis) in the form of a tea beverage for over one hundred years. The primary application has been for the treatment of the common cold and related respiratory symptoms. Independent reports by traditional herbalists on three Fijian islands invariably included strong, insistent statements that the decoction was very effective at treating head and chest congestion stemming from the common cold. As is typical with traditional medicines, efficacy for many other anti-microbial purposes was claimed. However, one key commonality across all herbalists was the application of the rhizome decoction for treatment of colds and related/similar symptoms. In order to achieve definitive outcomes, it was decided to promote and study the impact of Fijian Rhizophora solely on cold symptoms. Thus, the working hypothesis of our clinical self-report study was as follows:

A hot water decoction and/or specific glycerin-based fluidextract of Fijian Rhizophora mangle delivered via a fluidextract concentrate would produce a rapid (12-48 hours), significant, possibly complete, reduction of cold-related symptoms. (A previous study by Ted Anders, PhD. and reported to this researcher found the hypothesis to be supported with an observational sample of more than 60 clients ranging in age from 2-80.)

The pertinence of this clinical report study to the on-going assessment of traditional herbal medicinals around the world is significant in three ways. First, it is essential that all herbal medicinals, including Fijian Rhizophora mangle, receive scientific scrutiny to substantiate claims. Second, the knowledge base pertaining to Rhizophora mangle must be expanded and substantiated as there are historical reports and recent studies from around the globe indicating potential medicinal properties (Hernandez and Perez, 1978; Duke and Wain, 1981); including significant anti-viral properties (Premanathan, Arakaki, Izumi, et. al., 1999) . Third, in the case of Fijian Rhizophora, it appears the plants provide a unique, reliable, naturally occurring constituent combination which needs to be more thoroughly examined to identify the primary active constituent and other identified constituents as a broad spectrum, complimentary support to primary active constituent action. Such a contribution to the arsenal of health care supplements available to humanity would be useful and noteworthy.

METHODS
Selection and Description of Participants

During the 12-month time period from February, 2004 through February, 2005, Dr. Scott Carroll, M.D. conducted this initial clinical study focused on the "Fiji Titi /Fiji Tea " product created by Nature's Nurse, Inc. The patient sample included 84 patients between the ages of 3 and 74; male and female. These patients had 2 or more symptoms related to the common cold: nasal congestion; runny nose; sore throat; headache; cough (with or without chest congestion); and malaise.

TECHNICAL INFORMATION

The recommended protocol for product use was: 2 full droppers of concentrated fluidextract to 1 cup of water, 4 times daily (morning, noon, evening and bedtime) for two days.

The fluidextract concentrates used were of two types. One was a hot water decoction produced by Terradyne Naturale, Inc. in their laboratories located in Woodbine, Iowa. The concentrate was designed to equal the potency of the traditional dosage created from 50g of dried, crushed rhizome in 8 cups of water. The extraction was obtained with a hot water decoction, which produced a dark brown, thick liquid; the UV spectrum of which was ?280nm, Abs. 0.2972. The yield was 29 ml/100g from crushed, dried Rhizophora. The final concentration was 3.4g/ml (d~1.2) or 2ml/cup of water. This fluidextract requires the inclusion of a preservative, sodium benzoate, in the finished product. The delivery system was a 1 oz. brown actinic bottle with a 1 ml capacity dropper.

The second was a proprietary glycerin-base alcohol-free fluidextract, called a '3-3-6™' processed fluidextract, produced by Cedar Bear Naturales, Inc. at their central R&D/lab operations in Roosevelt, Utah. The 3-3-6™ process is a serialized technology designed to produce a finished fluid extract that equals or exceeds the efficacy of the traditional dosage created from 50g of dried, crushed rhizome in 8 cups of water. The 3-3-6™ fluid extraction results in a dark brown, high viscosity liquid, with a specific gravity of 1.190, and a 3-3-6™ standardized brix density of 53 (+/- 2%), The yield is based on a proprietary ml/g range of 29ml/Xg (noting that much less Rhizophora raw material is used in 3-3-6™ fluid extract process than that used for Terradyne hot water decoction) from crushed, dried Rhizophora. The 3-3-6™ fluid extract requires no preservative (or refrigeration after opening), even claiming a labeled shelf life of 3 years. The delivery system was a 1 oz brown actinic bottle with a 1 ml capacity dropper.

Approximately 50% of the patients received the Terradyne fluid extract and 50% the Cedar Bear fluid extract.

RESULTS

Of the 84 patients from whom this researcher was able to obtain a clinical report, the following results were obtained. Seventy nine percent (79%) of overall participants had either complete resolution of symptoms before or by the end of the 48 hour treatment period (the vast majority) or in those few remaining, significant improvement. Twenty one (21%) of the patients were not improved. Of significant note is that several of the patients with recurrent sinusitis were in the 79% group. These patients thereby avoided taking antibiotics; which more of them would have been apt to do, based on prior experience in this type of patient. These results were overall concomitant for both the 3-3-6™ fluidextract and water decoction preparations, though it was noted that some respondents reported when they used half the dose for the 3-3-6™ fluidextract they still obtained results concurrent with the standard prescribed dose for this study. This latter point begs the further question if a particular type of fluid extract preparation for Rhizophora also enhances and/or increases its efficacy and/or effectiveness, particularly where dose related factors are concerned.

DISCUSSION

There is clear evidence that the hypothesis was supported. The Fijian Rhizophora mangle (Fiji Titi) appears to be effective for the vast majority of clients within 48 hours. Even patients with resistant, recurring sinus infections who invariably wind up on an antibiotic experienced resolution of their symptoms. Of course, these results need to be replicated in a controlled, double-blind clinical trial. Nevertheless, the impact appears to be significant and should be stimulus for further research.

The immediate implication for clinical practitioners is simple. At the onset of a cold or within 24 hours, Fijian Rhizophora mangle (Fiji Titi /Fiji Tea) in the concentrated fluid extract delivery systems created by Nature's Nurse, Inc. is a valuable, effective treatment. (The raw root tea is also effective but not the preferred delivery system by the vast majority of clients.) There were no reported, adverse side effects for any participant of any age in this study or that conducted by Ted Anders, PhD. and reported to this researcher. As the village herbalists informed Dr. Anders at the beginning of his research in 1998, this gentle, traditional medicinal rhizome appears to be appropriate for all ages from toddlers through senior adults.

REFERENCES

Duke, J.A. and K.K. Wain, *Medicinal Plants of the World*, 3 Volumes, 1981.

Hernandez N. M. Rojas and Coto O. Perez, "Antimicrobial properties of extracts from Rhizophora mangle," *Rev. Cubana Med Trop* 30 (1978): 181-187.

Premanathan, N., Kathiresan, K., Yamamoto, N., Nakashima, H., "In-vitro anti-human immunodeficiency virus activity of polysaccharide from Rhizophora mucronata poir," *Biosci, Biotechnol, Biochem* 63 (1999): 1187-91.

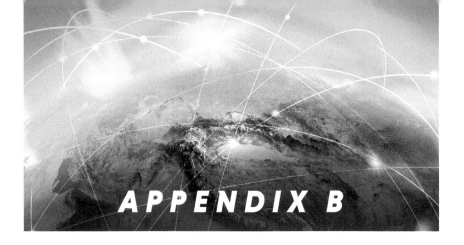

APPENDIX B

RESEARCH ARTICLES IN SUPPORT OF RESPIGARD™ EFFICACY: RESPIRATORY & IMMUNE SYSTEM SUPPORT

(Respigard ™ Active Ingredient: Rhizophora mangle L. in a base of vegetable glycerin)

THE GLOBAL RESEARCH ON THE EFFECTS OF red mangrove extracts and some of its primary active phtyochemical compounds is extensive. A synthesis of a subset of the research can be summarized as follows:

"The phytochemical constituents and whole component parts of red mangrove (Rhizpophora mangle, L.) are known to provide anti-microbial, anti-inflammatory, immune-modulating, anti-pyretic, and anti-oxidant functions. Some of the primary constituents are Complex Polysaccharide Compounds, Salicylates, and Polyphenols & Phytosterols including specified tannic acids and members of the sub-class of polyphenols known as Flavonoids: Quercitin, Umbelliferone (7-hydroxycoumarin), Luteolin, Kaempferol, and Isorhamnetin ."

Ted D. Anders, Ph.D.

The FDA-compliant botanical structure/function statement for Respigard™:

"Supports Respiratory and Immune Systems Function... ...during Seasonal and Ongoing Challenges"

Research Bibliography (presented by general metabolic activity) Upper Respiratory Infection References

1. Carroll, Scott , "The effect of Fijian Red Mangrove (Rhizophora mangle) on the common cold," Atlanta Allergy & Asthma Institute and Nature's Nurse, Inc., published online January 5, 2006, www.naturesnurse.com/research, 1-4.
2. Doseff, A. I., Arango, D., Cardenas, H. Nicholas, C.,Nuova, G., Grotewold, E., "Thematic Poster Session—Novel Therapeutic Options in Airways Disease," *American Journal of Respiratory and Critical Care Medicine* (2011).
3. Heinz, S.A., Henson, D.A., Austin, M.D., Jin, F., Nieman, D.C., "Quercitin supplementation and upper respiratory tract infection: A randomized clinical trial," *Pharmacological Research* 62(3): 237-242.

4. Trivedi, R., Anders, T.D., et. al., "The effect of red mangrove aqueous extract (Rhizopphora mangle, L.) on Upper Respiratory Tract Infections (URTI)," published online April, 2012, by Nature's Nurse International, Inc., www.naturesnurse.com/research.

5. Yi, L., Li, Z., et al, "Small molecules blocking the entry of severe acute respiratory syndrome coronavirus into host cells," *Journal of Virology* (2004): 11334-11339.

Immune System Modulation References

6. Chunchao, H., Guo, J., "A hypothesis: supplementation with mushroom-derived active hexose correlated compound modulates immunity and increases survival in response to influenza virus (H1N1) infection," *Evidence-Based Complementary and Alternative Medicine* (2011): 1-3.

7. Reynolds, J.A., Kastello, M.D., Harrington, D. G., Crabbs, C.L., Peters, C. J., Jemenksi, J.V., Scott, G.H., Di Luzio, N.R., "Glucan-induced enhancement of host resistance to selected infectious diseases," *Infection and Immunity* (1980): 51-57.

8. Ritz, B.W., Nogusa, S., Ackerman, E. A., Gardner, E., "Supplementation with active hexose correlated compound increases the innate immune response of young mice to primary influenza infection," *American Society for Nutrition* (2006): 2868-2873.

9. Ritz, B. W., 2011, "Fermented mushroom extract affects immune outcomes and immune cell populations," *Enzyme Science*, published online Jan 1, 2011, 1-7.

10. Spierlings, L.H. E., Fujii, H., Buxiang, S., Walshe, T., "A phase study of the safety of the nutritional supplement, active hexose

correlated compound, AHCC, in healthy volunteers," *Journal of Nutritional Science and Vitaminology*, 53 (2007): 536-539.

11. Tzianabos, A., O., "Polysaccharide immunomodulators as therapeutic agents: structural aspects and biologic function," *Clinical Microbiology Reviews* (2000): 523-533.

Anti-Microbial Constituent References and Mangrove Component References

12. Basile. A., Giordano, S., Lopez-Saez, J.A., Cobianchi, R. C., "Antibacterial activity of pure flavonoids isolated from mosses," *Phytochemistry* 52 (1999):1479-1482.

13. Chandrasekaran, M., Kannathasan, K., Venkatesalu, V., Prabhakar, K., "Antibacterial activity of some salt marsh halophytes and mangrove plants against methicillin resistant Stapholococcus aureus," published online October, 2008, Springer-Science + Business Media B.V.

14. de Armas, E., Sarracent, Y., Marrero, E., Fernandez, O., Branford-White, C., "Efficacy of Rhizophora mangle aqueous bark extract (RMABE) in the treatment of apthous ulcers: a pilot study," *Current Medical Research and Opinion* 21(11) (2006): 1711-1715.

15. Hicks, M., Bailey, M.A., Thiagarajan, T.R., Troyer, T. L., Huggins, L.G., "Antibacterial and Cytotoxic Effects of Red Mangrove (Rhizophora Mangle L. Rhizophoraceae) Fruit Extract," *European Journal of Scientific Research* 63(3) (2011): 439-446.

16. Lyu,S., Rhim, J., Park, W., "Antiherpetic activities of flavonoids against herpes simplex virus type 1 (HSV-1) and type 2 (HSV-2) in vitro," *Archives of Pharmacology Research* 28/11 (2005): 1293-1301.

17. Melchor, G., Armenteros, M., Fernández, O., Linares, E., Fragas, I., "Antibacterial activity of Rhizophora mangle bark," *Fitoterapia* 72 (6) (2001): 689-691.
18. Ravikumar, S., Inbaneson, S. J., Suganthi, P., Venkatesan, M., and Ramu, A., "Mangrove plants as a source of lead compounds for the development of antiplasmodal drugs from South East coast of India", *Parasitol Research* 108 (2011): 1405-1410.
19. Sanchez Perera, M.L., Varcalcel, L., Escobar, A., Noa, M., "Polyphenol and Phytosterol Composition in an Antibacterial Extract from Rhizophora mangle," L. Bark, *Journal of Herbal Pharmacotherapy*, 7(3-4) (2007).
20. Tsai, F., Lin, C., Lai, C., Lan, L., Lai, C., Hung, C., Hsueh, K., Lin, T., Chang, H., Wan, L., Jinn-Chyuan Sheu, J., and Ying-Ju Lin. "Kaempferol inhibits enterovirus 71 replication and internal ribosome entry site (IRES) activity through FUBP and HNRP proteins," *Food Chemistry* 128(2) (2011): 312-322.

Anti-Inflammatory Constituent References

21. Calderón-Montaño, J., Burgos-Morón, E., Pérez-Guerrero, C. and M. López-Lázaro, "A Review on the Dietary Flavonoid Kaempferol," *Mini-Reviews in Medicinal Chemistry* 11 (2011): 298-344.
22. Cho, S., Park, S., Kwon,M., Jeong,T., Bok, S., Choi, W., Jeong, W., Ryu, S., Do, S., Lee, C., Song, J., Jeong, K. "Quercetin suppresses proinflammatory cytokine production through MAP kinases and NF-κBpathway in lipopolysaccharide-stimulated macrophage," *Molecular and Cellular Biochemistry* 243 (2003): 153–160.

23. Courtney, N., 2012, "The anti-inflammatory mechanisms of the flavonoid apigenin in vitro and in vivo," OhioLINK ETD Center, July 2012, http://rave.ohiolink.edu/etdc/view?acc_num=osu1259783472, 1-2.

24. García-Mediavilla, V., Crespo, I., Collado, P., Esteller, A., Sánchez-Campos, S., Tuñón, M., González-Gallego, J. "The anti-inflammatory flavones quercetin and kaempferol cause inhibition of inducible nitric oxide synthase, cyclooxygenase-2 and reactive C-protein, and down-regulation of the nuclear factor kappaB pathway in Chang Liver cells," *European Journal of Pharmacology* 557(2-3) (2007):221-229.

25. Jang, S., Kelley, K., and R. W. Johnson. "Luteolin reduces IL-6 production in microglia by inhibiting JNK phosphorylation and activation of AP-1," *Proceedings of the National Academy of Sciences* 105(21) (2008): 7534-7539.

26. Karlsem, A., Rettersol, L., Laake, P., Paur, I., Kjolsrud-Bohn, S., Sandvik, L., Blomhoff, R, "Anthocyanins inhibit nuclear factor-kB activation in monocytes and reduce plasma concentrations of pro-inflammatory mediators in healthy adults," *Journal of Nutrition* 137 (2007): 1951-1954.

27. Kelly, G. S., Quercetin Monograph, *Alternative Medicine Review* 16(2) (2011): 172-194.

28. Lino, C. S., Taveira, M. L., Vianaw, G. S. B., and F. J. A. Matos. "Analgesic and Anti-inflammatory Activities of *Justicia pectoralis* Jacq and its Main Constituents: Coumarin and Umbelliferone," *Phytotherapy Research*, 11 (1997): 211–215.

29. López-Lázaro, M. "Distribution and Biological Activities of the Flavonoid Luteolin," *Mini-Reviews in Medicinal Chemistry* 9 (2009): 31-59.

30. Nicholas, C., Batra, S., Vargo, M. A., Voss, O. H., Gavrilin, M. A., Wewers, M.D., Guttridge, D.C., Grotewold, E., Doseff,

A.I., "Apigenin blocks lipopolysaccharide-induced lethality in vivo and proinflammatory cytokines expression by inactivating NF-kB through suppression of p65 phosphorylation," *The Journal of Immunology* 179: 7121-7127.

31. Taís A. de Almeida Barrosa, Luis A.R. de Freitasa, José M.B. Filhob, Xirley P. Nunesb, Ana M. Giuliettic, Glória E. de Souzad, Ricardo R. dos Santosa,e, Milena B.P. Soaresa,e and Cristiane F. Villarreal, "Antinociceptive and anti-inflammatory properties of 7-hydroxycoumarin in experimental animal models: potential therapeutic for the control of inflammatory chronic pain," *Journal of Pharmacy and Pharmacology* 62 (2010): 205–213.

32. Theoharides, T. "Luteolin as a therapeutic option for multiple sclerosis," *Journal of Neuroinflammation* 6 (2009): 29-31.

33. Yoon,J., Lee, H., Choi, S., Chang, E., Lee, S., Lee, E. "Quercetin Inhibits IL-1b-Induced Inflammation, Hyaluronan Production and Adipogenesis in Orbital Fibroblasts from Graves' Orbitopathy," *PLos ONE* 6(10) (2011): 1-10.

Anti-Oxidant Constituent References

34. Berenguer, B., Sanchez, L.M., Quilez, A., Lopez-Barreiro, M., de Haro, O., Galvez, J., and Martin, M. J., "Protective and Antioxidant effects of Rhizophora mangle, L. against NSAID-induced gastric ulcers," *Journal of Ethno-Pharmacology* 103 (2006), 194-200.

35. Fabiani, R., Rosignoli, P., De Bartolomeo, A., Fuccelli, R., Servili, M., Montedoro, G. F., Morozzi, G., "Oxidative DNA damage is prevented by extracts of olive oil, hydroxytyrosol, and other olive phenolic compounds in human blood mono-

nuclear cells and HL60 cells," *Journal of Nutrition* 138 (2008): 1411-1416.

36. Sánchez,J., Melchor, G., Martínez, G., Escobar, A., Faure, R., "Antioxidant activity of Rhizophora mangle bark," *Fitoterapia*, Vol. 77, Issue 2 (2006): 141-143.

37. Sanchez, M., Lodi, F., Vera, R., Villar, C., Cogolludo, A., Jimenez, R., Moreno, L., Romero, M., Tamargo, J., Perez-Vizcaino, F., and J. Duarte, "Quercetin and Isorhamnetin Prevent Endothelial Dysfunction, Superoxide Production, and Overexpression of p47phox Induced by Angiotensin II in Rat Aorta1," *Journal of Nutrition* 137 (2007): 910–915.

38. Zielińska, M., Kostrzewa, A., Ignatowicz, E., and J. Budzianowski, "The flavonoids, quercetin and isorhamnetin 3-O-acylglucosides diminish neutrophil oxidative metabolism and lipid peroxidation," *Acta Biochimica Polonica* 48(1) (2001): 183-189.

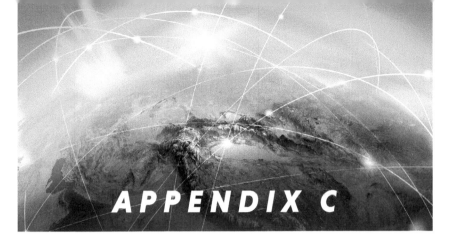

APPENDIX C

RESEARCH ARTICLES IN
SUPPORT OF SKINGARD™
EFFICACY

**(Skingard ™ Active Ingredient: Rhizophora mangle L.
in a base of vegetable glycerin)**

THE GLOBAL RESEARCH ON THE EFFECTS OF red mangrove extracts
and some of its primary active phtyochemical compounds on skin
health is extensive. A synthesis of the research can be summarized in
the following FDA-compliant statement:

"Botanical Structure/Function Statement:
Skingard™ Supports Healthy Skin Tissue ..."
The product is used during a variety of minor accidental, post-surgical,
environmental, and natural challenges to skin health ... while also providing anti-oxidants which are known to provide anti-aging support.

Dr. Ted Anders

Research Bibliography

1. Berenguer, B., Sanchez, L.M., Quilez, A., Lopez-Barreiro, M., de Haro, O., Galvez, J., and Martin, M. J., "Protective and Antioxidant effects of Rhizophora mangle, L. against NSAID-induced gastric ulcers," *Journal of Ethno-Pharmacology* 103 (2006): 194-200.

2. Chandrasekaran, M., Kannathasan, K., Venkatesalu, V., Prabhakar, K "Antibacterial activity of some salt marsh halpophytes and mangrove plants against methicillin resistant Stapholococcus aureus," Springer-Science + Business Media B.V., published online October 19, 2008.

3. Cho, S., Park, S., Kwon,M., Jeong,T., Bok, S., Choi, W., Jeong, W., Ryu, S., Do, S., Lee, C., Song, J., Jeong, K, "Quercetin suppresses proinflammatory cytokine production through MAP kinases and NF-κBpathway in lipopolysaccharide-stimulated macrophage," *Molecular and Cellular Biochemistry* 243:(2003):153–160.

4. de Armas, E., Sarracent, Y., Marrero, E., Fernandez, O., Branford-White, C., "Efficacy of Rhizophora mangle aqueous bark extract (RMABE) in the treatment of apthous ulcers: a pilot study," *Current Medical Research and Opinion* 21(11) (2006): 1711-1715.

5. Fernandez, O., Capdevila, J. Z., Dalla, G., Melchor, G., " Efficacy of Rhizophora mangle aqueous bark extract in the healing of open surgical wounds," *Fitoterapia* Vol. 73, Issues 7–8 (2002): 564-568.

6. Gleiby Melchor, Mabelin Armenteros, Octavio Fernández, Eliana Linares, Ivis Fragas, "Antibacterial activity of Rhizophora mangle bark," *Fitoterapia* Vol. 72, Issue 6 (2001): 689-691.

7. Hicks, M., Bailey, M.A., Thiagarajan, T.R., Troyer, T. L., Huggins, L.G., "Antibacterial and Cytotoxic Effects of Red Mangrove (Rhizophora Mangle L. Rhizophoraceae) Fruit Extract," *European Journal of Scientific Research* 63(3) (2011): 439-446.

8. Kelly, G. S., Quercetin Monograph, *Alternative Medicine Review* 16(2) (2011):172-194.

9. List, R., Patent Application Document, Application Number: EP2010/053096. An adhesive patch according to any one of claims 2 and 4, wherein said at least one therapeutic agent comprises red mangrove. (Herpes treatment), 2011.

10. Lyu, S., Rhim, J., Park, W., "Antiherpetic activities of flavonoids against herpes simplex virus type 1 (HSV-1) and type 2 (HSV-2) in vitro, *Archives of Pharmacology Research* 28/11 (2005): 1293-1301.

11. Marrero, E., Sánchez, J., de Armas, E., Escobar, A., Melchor, G., Abad, M.J., Bermejo, P., Villar, A.M., Megías, J., Alcaraz, M.J., "COX-2 and sPLA₂ inhibitory activity of aqueous extract and polyphenols of Rhizophora mangle (red mangrove)," *Fitoterapia* Vol. 77, Issue 4, (2006): 313-315.

12. Meira de-Faria, F., Alves Almeida, A.C., Luiz-Ferreira, A., Dunder, R.J., Takayama,C., Silene da Silva, M., Aparecido da Silva, M., Vilegas, W., Rozza, A. L., Pellizzon, C. H., Toma, W., Monteiro Souza-Brito, A.G., "Mechanisms of action underlying the gastric antiulcer activity of the Rhizophora mangle L.," *Journal of Ethnopharmacology* Vol. 139, Issue 1 (2012): 234-243.

13. Sánchez, J., Melchor, G., Martínez, G., Escobar, A., Faure, R., Antioxidant activity of Rhizophora mangle bark," *Fitoterapia* Vol. 77, Issue 2 (2006) : 141-143.

14. Sanchez Perera, M.L., Varcalcel, L., Escobar, A., Noa, M., "Polyphenol and Phytosterol Composition in an Antibacterial

Extract from Rhizophora mangle, L. Bark," *Journal of Herbal Pharmacotherapy*, Vol. 7 (2007): 3-4.

15. Vu Huong Giang, Le Quynh Lien, Ninh Khac Ban, Chau Van Minh, "Evaluation of Bacteria Inhibitory Activity of Mangrove Flora in Xuan Thuy National Park," *Bio Magazine* 35-3 (2013): 342-347

Research Relevant to Wounds & Lesions

1. Berenguer, B., Sanchez, L.M., Quilez, A., Lopez-Barreiro, M., de Haro, O., Galvez, J., and Martin, M. J., "Protective and Antioxidant effects of Rhizophora mangle, L. against NSAID-induced gastric ulcers," *Journal of Ethno-Pharmacology* 103 (2006): 194-200.

2. Chandrasekaran, M., Kannathasan, K., Venkatesalu, V., Prabhakar, K., published online October 19, 2008, "Antibacterial activity of some salt marsh halpophytes and mangrove plants against methicillin resistant Stapholococcus aureus," Springer-Science + Business Media B.V.

3. Cho, S., Park, S., Kwon, M., Jeong, T., Bok, S., Choi, W., Jeong, W., Ryu, S., Do, S., Lee, C., Song, J., Jeong, K., "Quercetin suppresses proinflammatory cytokine production through MAP kinases and NF-κBpathway in lipopolysaccharide-stimulated macrophage." *Molecular and Cellular Biochemistry* 243 (2003): 153–160.

4. de Armas, E., Sarracent, Y., Marrero, E., Fernandez, O., Branford-White, C, "Efficacy of Rhizophora mangle aqueous bark extract (RMABE) in the treatment of apthous ulcers: a pilot study," *Current Medical Research and Opinion* 21(11) (2006): 1711-1715.

5. Fernandez, O., J.Z Capdevila, G Dalla, G Melchor, "Efficacy of Rhizophora mangle aqueous bark extract in the healing of open surgical wounds," *Fitoterapia* Vol. 73, Issues 7–8 (2002): 564-568.

6. Gleiby Melchor, Mabelin Armenteros, Octavio Fernández, Eliana Linares, Ivis Fragas, "Antibacterial activity of Rhizophora mangle bark," *Fitoterapia* Vol. 72, Issue 6 (2001): 689-691.

7. Hicks, M., Bailey, M.A., Thiagarajan, T.R., Troyer, T. L., Huggins, L.G "Antibacterial and Cytotoxic Effects of Red Mangrove (Rhizophora Mangle L. Rhizophoraceae) Fruit Extract," *European Journal of Scientific Research*, 63(3) (2011): 439-446.

8. Kelly, G. S., Quercetin Monograph, *Alternative Medicine Review* 16(2) (2011):172-194.

9. List, R., Patent Application Document, Application Number: EP2010/053096. An adhesive patch according to any one of claims 2 and 4, wherein said at least one therapeutic agent comprises red mangrove (Herpes treatment), 2011.

10. Lyu,S., Rhim, J., Park, W., "Antiherpetic activities of flavonoids against herpes simplex virus type 1 (HSV-1) and type 2 (HSV-2) in vitro," *Archives of Pharmacology Research*, 28/11 (2005): 1293-1301.

11. Marrero, Evangelina, Janet Sánchez, Elizabeth de Armas, Arturo Escobar, Gleiby Melchor, M.J. Abad, Paulina Bermejo, Angel M. Villar, J. Megías, Maria J. Alcaraz, "COX-2 and sPLA2 inhibitory activity of aqueous extract and polyphenols of Rhizophora mangle (red mangrove)," Fitoterapia Vol. 77, Issue 4 (2006): 313-315.

12. Meira de-Faria, Felipe, Ana Cristina Alves Almeida, Anderson Luiz-Ferreira, Ricardo José Dunder, Christiane Takayama, Maria Silene da Silva, Marcelo Aparecido da Silva, Wagner Vilegas, Ariane Leite Rozza, Cláudia Helena Pellizzon, Walber

Toma, Alba Regina Monteiro Souza-Brito, "Mechanisms of action underlying the gastric antiulcer activity of the Rhizophora mangle L.," *Journal of Ethnopharmacology* Vol. 139, Issue 1 (2012): 234-243.

13. Odio, A. D., Gonzalez, J. E., Sanchez, M. L., Delgado, N. G., "Genotoxic assessment of aqueous extract of Rhizophora mangle L. (mangle rojo) by spermatozoa head assay," published online: http://bvs.sld.cu/revistas/pla/vol_15_1_10/pla03110.htm.

14. Sánchez, Janet, Gleiby Melchor, Gregorio Martínez, Arturo Escobar, Roberto Faure. "Antioxidant activity of Rhizophora mangle bark," Fitoterapia Vol. 77, Issue 2 (2006): 141-143.

15. Sanchez Perera, M.L., Varcalcel, L., Escobar, A., Noa, M., "Polyphenol and Phytosterol Composition in an Antibacterial Extract from Rhizophora mangle, L. Bark," *Journal of Herbal Pharmacotherapy*, Vol. 7 (3-4) (2007).

ABOUT THE AUTHORS

Ted Anders, PhD

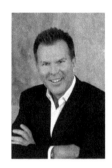

Ted was born in Norfolk, Virginia to a minister father and school teacher mother who taught him the values and joy of service to humanity. His educational and humanitarian interests have always been wide ranging. After graduating from Furman University with a degree in Pscyhology, he served as a volunteer mission teacher in an American Quaker high school in Ramallah, Palestine to promote peace among Palestinians and Israelis. Ted met and married Grace Janho in Jerusalem, with whom he has two daughters, Hannah and Natalie, who reside in California.

He continued his psychology studies at the University of Georgia where he earned MS and PhD degrees in Educational Psychology, with a focus on human learning and performance. Following his formal education, Ted shaped a career which allowed him to continue exploring the world and beyond. He became an Astronaut Training Manager at NASA's Johnson Space Center and then went on to advise aerospace firms, the US military, businesses, school systems and hospitals on management systems which value and stimulate the best in all employees. His proprietary management system, known as "Customer Driven Leadership," has been applied on five continents from 1995 to the present.

During 25 years as a consultant, Ted traveled around the globe many times serving his clients. While on these travels, he began exploring the natural traditional medicines of the South Pacific. He met co-author Resina Koroi and together they "re-discovered" the powerful traditional medicines derived from red mangrove. He created the Nature's Nurse companies in the US and Fiji to harvest, research, develop, and market these botanical resources in an ecologically sustainable manner, while honoring the indigenous culture and economic development goals of the Fijian people.

Ted's interests are now focused on assisting people around the world to improve their health and wellness naturally. He believes when people get well using natural products, their concerns for protecting and reclaiming Earth's damaged ecosystems will increase. In fact, his companies implement the doctrine promoted by an investor in the Nature's Nurse companies, "The World Restored, Not Destroyed." He shares the concerns of Jean-Michel Cousteau and his Ocean Futures Society that humans must immediately take action to protect and preserve our oceans, shoreline ecosystems, and the rest of Earth. After all, pollution from land-based activities makes its way inexorably into the oceans via runoff into our streams and rivers. Now is the time for us all to wake up and recognize humans and the Earth are completely interdependent and we must nurture nature if we want to thrive here for generations to come.

Resina Koroi

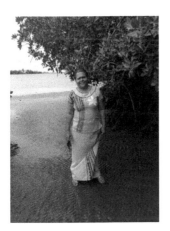

Resina Koroi, the co-founder of Nature's Nurse Fiji, Ltd., and Nature's Nurse International, Inc., is a strong advocate of women's issues at the grassroots level in the community. Volunteering for four years at a school for marginalized children with special needs, she was faced with the daily challenges they faced from home. Eighty percent of these children came from single parent families and families who had migrated to the city in search of better opportunities.

In 2005, Resina became a Rotarian and took on the Rotary projects to help the community. The first major project Resina embarked on was the construction and opening of Fiji's first ever dialysis centre for kidney disease patients. Up until 2007, patients diagnosed with kidney disease needing dialysis or treatment had to spend their own money to travel to New Zealand, Australia or India for treatment. With the opening of the Fiji dialysis centre, these patients could have treatment locally and remain with their families.

In 2007, a group of Rotarians approached Resina to complete a proposal for a 3H Grant from Rotary to fund water projects in Fiji and for her to head the project. The grant was successful for USD$300, 000 and the Rotary Pacific Water for Life Foundation was formed. Partnering with local organizations, USD$ 1.5 million dollars was raised to implement the two-year project.

The first year was spent conducting community visitations, evaluations and the creation of a framework for the timely and efficient delivery of the water project with the relevant stakeholders. By the second year 150 water projects were completed throughout Fiji.

During this time, Resina worked with local non-government organizations, provincial councils, government ministries, diplomatic missions and other civic-minded citizens to achieve the Foundation's goal of providing safe drinking water to needy communities throughout Fiji.

Resina also worked for the country's national airline in the late 80's to early 2003 as a flight attendant and completed her career for Air Pacific as a purser and trainer.

Resina has been described by the people she has worked with as "the person that makes things happen" and she will always find a way to surmount the impossible.

NOTES